Praise For Making Wellbeing Practical

"Using a personable voice that is easy to connect with, this book offers practical ways for supporting student wellbeing. Luke offers background and rationale for the concepts building on research from the wellbeing sciences, combined with practical approaches for application."

Associate Professor Peggy Kern, PhD, Centre for Positive Psychology, The University of Melbourne's Graduate School of Education (creator of the PERMAH Workplace and EPOCH surveys, accessible at www.peggykern.org)

"Luke McKenna is passionate about helping schools and young people to thrive. In his book, *Making Wellbeing Practical*, Luke shares his considerable knowledge of the growing field of wellbeing science and then shares a range of personal wellbeing practices that are practical and engaging for young people. This book is a valuable addition to the field and provides educators with a strong foundational knowledge of wellbeing, increasing the likelihood for the successful implementation of placing wellbeing at the heart of our schools."

Justin Robinson- Director- Institute of Positive Education- Geelong Grammar School

"I have had the privilege of working with Luke McKenna and his team from UPP since he made the decision to take leave from his Assistant Principal role and begin UPP, in order to increase growth mindsets, grit, well-being and leadership capacity in students right across the country. Students at Marist College Ashgrove now look forward to "their turn" to work with the UPP team as they have seen and heard of the impact they have.

Now that Luke has written *Making Wellbeing Practical,* we have an opportunity to bring his voice into the school on a regular basis. More importantly though is the security of knowing that this voice is evidence-based, well-researched and tried and tested through personal experience. This will build a sense of confidence in the teachers delivering the PWPs from the book; knowing what they are facilitating with our students is part of a much bigger picture, based on the well proven tenets of Positive Psychology.

Bruce McPhee- Deputy Headmaster- Marist College, Ashgrove

"As you delve into *Making Wellbeing Practical* you'll quickly realise that Luke McKenna really knows his stuff! This book has translated deep understandings into real-life practical tools that can be applied in schools to improve student wellbeing. Making Wellbeing Practical is a tremendous resource for any school leader wanting to know and understand wellbeing and positive education and how to implement it successfully in their school."

James Anderson- Speaker, Author, Educator- Mindful by Design

"Luke's offering was a breath of fresh air for the Wellbeing and Positive Education space. It was quickly apparent early in the book that Luke has completed comprehensive research in the area and has got his head around it. Luke put meat on the bones of many the tenets and rationales that we operate (or should operate) schools by through logical, extensive and well documented research findings. His experience as a leader at the coalface in schools added immense credibility to what he wrote, and quite frankly, made the research vindicate what great teachers have been doing for years, educating the whole child. It was Luke's reading between the lines of research which impressed me most. Often research is a cold and distant pursuit and its findings quite difficult to apply in schools. Luke eloquently overcame this for me. Practitioners in schools will readily be able to understand and implement the raft of ideas and strategies he has presented in the book.

His efforts to use humour to lighten and brighten up the words for the reader were also much appreciated. I would highly recommend Luke's book as a great read and valuable resource to underpin any Wellbeing / Positive Education courses that you may have in your school."
Mick Walsh- Author, Educator, Speaker- The Learning Curve

"Luke McKenna's energy and enthusiasm for supporting wellbeing in schools comes across loudly and clearly in his new book. *Making Wellbeing Practical* provides a clear and comprehensive overview of the elements of wellbeing defined in Martin Seligman's popular PERMA(H) model. In addition, it offers a plethora of activities and ideas designed to help students develop their wellbeing skills. Anyone interested in bringing PERMAH based wellbeing strategies into their school will find this book a rich and indispensable guide."
Dr Helen Street, Applied Social Psychologist, Founder: The Positive Schools Initiative

"After reading *Making Wellbeing Practical*, I can't wait to get it into our school! To be able to support staff and student wellbeing through the knowledge gained and the practices that build wealth will be invaluable. The Personal Wellbeing Practices seamlessly tie in to our weekly PB4L focus, and will help our community to thrive!"
Michelle Heather- Primary Learning Leader- St Thomas More School, Sunshine Beach

"*Making Wellbeing Practical* is an enjoyable and thought provoking read that integrates evidence with a range of personal experiences within the classroom and other real life situations. The suggested strategies provide a blueprint for embedding wellbeing and positive education within our school setting, while its practical suggestions help to cultivate a wellbeing mindset in our everyday lives."

Peter Groundwater- Deputy Principal- St Teresa's Catholic College, Abergowrie

"Luke's book is very well done. It is the perfect combination of research, theory and practice. This book is clear and concise and offers much more information than I expected. I have and will continue to share UPP's work in all levels of education. I encourage every educator to read, engage and apply *Making Wellbeing Practical.*"

Clint Curran- Principal- Runaway Bay Sport & Leadership Excellence Centre

"I will be sure to get a copy for all teachers, middle and senior leaders of wellbeing in our College. *Making Wellbeing Practical* is not only a good resource for educators but for families who want to understand their children more."

Mark Kennedy- Deputy Principal (Senior Years)- St Joseph's College, Geelong

"Once again Luke and his team have delivered another terrific resource for our students based on well-founded research mixed with real life experiences. This book provides schools with excellent resources that you can implement very easily and has such lasting impact on the lives of our young people. Definitely a must have resource in reducing the growing tide of mental health issues in our community for years to come."

Nick Antoniazzi- Deputy Principal (Student Services)- St Anthony's Catholic College, Townsville

"*Making Wellbeing Practical* unpacks Wellbeing and Positive Education in a practical and logical way for educators. The Personal Wellbeing Practices will greatly assist teachers to embed the PERMAH pillars and make it doable in classrooms."

Belinda Ryan- Deputy Principal and Student Wellbeing Leader- Our Lady of the Rosary, Kyneton

MAKING WELLBEING PRACTICAL

AN EFFECTIVE GUIDE TO HELPING SCHOOLS THRIVE

LUKE MCKENNA

UNLEASHING PERSONAL POTENTIAL

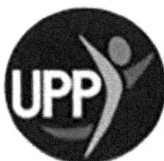

unleashingpersonalpotential.com.au

First published in Australia 2019
Copyright © 2019 Luke McKenna

Prepublication Data Services available on request from the National Library of Australia.

ISBN: 978-0-9943866-1-8 (pbk)

Edited by Gayle Oddy

Typesetting and design by Publicious P/L
www.publicious.com.au

Published with the assistance of Publicious P/L
www.publicious.com.au

TABLE OF CONTENTS

Positive Emotion

ABOUT UNLEASHING PERSONAL POTENTIAL (UPP)

At UPP, our mission is for every student to become the best they can be. Our vision is to impact 50,000 students each year to LEARN, LIVE AND LEAD better, through exceptional incursions.

UPP specialises in making Wellbeing and Positive Education practical. We do this by making scientifically grounded strategies engaging, relevant, challenging and inspiring for schools.

We deliver exceptional student incursions and camps; engaging, relevant, practical online lesson plans; and high quality professional development for teachers.

We seek to live and work by the values of excellence, character and contribution.

In 2018, we impacted 30,000+ students to LEARN, LIVE AND LEAD better, through exceptional incursions.

ABOUT THE AUTHOR

LUKE MCKENNA

UPP Founder and Director, Luke McKenna, is an educator and author who specialises in working with schools to help students learn, live and lead better. He has worked as a classroom teacher, middle school leader and Assistant Principal, before founding UPP in 2015. Luke has worked with educators and students across Australian primary and secondary schools from the independent, Catholic and public sectors.

He holds degrees in Business and Education, a Masters of Educational Leadership and a Professional Certificate in Positive Education.

Luke regularly speaks at conferences around Australia. His work has been published in the Australian Journal of Middle Schooling, Happy Schools and The Positive Times, and he is also the author of 'Thrive: Unlocking the truth about student performance'.

ABOUT THE CONTRIBUTING AUTHOR

LAURA MCKENNA

Laura McKenna is a Registered Nurse, author and instructor of Yoga, Meditation and Wellbeing. After more than a decade in the health industry in a number of roles in hospitals and community nursing, Laura has identified a huge need for proactive wellbeing strategies. Recently, Laura has been developing many of UPP's Personal Wellbeing Practices and brings a health professional's perspective to Wellbeing and Positive Education.

Laura and Luke live in Brisbane with their three gorgeous kids – Elijah, Oscar and Ava.

A NOTE OF GRATITUDE

Four years after beginning Unleashing Personal Potential, I am grateful.

I am grateful to have worked with some of Australia's best educators. I am inspired by their contribution, passion and desire to make the world a better place through education.

I'm grateful to be able to lead a team of passionate educators. Their positivity, humour and zest make this work so enjoyable.

We now have the opportunity to work with people all over this amazing country and to do meaningful work. Our vision for UPP was initially much smaller than it is right now. I am grateful to every educator in our partner schools who gave us an opportunity to work with their students, before we really knew what we were doing! We are still (and ever will be) working it out!

This book has been influenced by the work of many amazing people.
- Researchers and thought leaders (most of whom I have never met, some of whom I call friends).
- Our fantastic pre-readers who willingly provided wonderful feedback and comments to help make this book better for our readers.
- Justin Robinson, Mick Walsh, James Anderson, Helen Street and Peggy Kern- who were able to provide genuine insight and

perspective on this work. Your feedback has been invaluable to the process of making this book the best it can be.

- Members of our production team. Gayle Oddy- our editor, who spent countless hours proofreading and editing this work. Andy at Publicious Pty Ltd for his support and guidance in the publishing process. Sam and Bhanuka- our graphic designers- because at times, a picture is worth 1000 words.

- Our amazing team at UPP, in particular Hogan Rogers and Pete McAuliffe, who have stepped up to challenges beyond their years and who show maturity, along with a huge commitment to our values of character, excellence and contribution. It has been amazing to watch each of you grow. I am convinced that you will continue to make significant contributions, both professionally and personally. You have stepped up and it has been a pleasure to observe your growth.

On a more personal note…

To my mum and dad and my brothers and sisters. What an opportunity it was growing up in a home with so much love, care and support from each of you. Sorry that I came along instead of the pool you were meant to get! Despite that, each of you has offered so much to my life and I hope that I can somehow repay you for the contribution, example and perspective you have brought to mine. You are all amazing people and so are your partners and kids. Once again, credit to Mum and Dad for that.

I'm grateful to my beautiful wife, Laura. For your enduring support of this (sometimes obsessive) passion. For getting on board. For telling me when I'm probably wrong. For love. For accepting me as I am and challenging me to be better. For riding the highs and lows with me and being able to provide much perspective and insight along the way. For late nights when you didn't really want to be talking about work. For the many hours you spent bringing our PWP's to life. Thank you.

I'm so grateful to have been blessed with three kids. I love each of you so very much. I'd love to be a perfect dad, but I'm grateful that you love me when I'm not. I'm grateful that I get to invest my life in you and help you be the best people you can.

INTRODUCTION

I've always had an interest in self-improvement. Ever since I can remember, I've been intrigued by certain people who seem to have made their lives work better than most others. My dad is a good example of someone like this. He had a somewhat unfortunate upbringing – after being disowned by his parents for no good reason he was raised by his aunty and uncle. He had a lot to complain about. He could have become resentful. He is now one of the most loving men I know. He doesn't say much, but he shows a lot of love and he holds his family and friends very close. He could have gone the other way, but he chose how to respond.

Some people rise – and some collapse. It always fascinated me, but I could always empathise and see both sides. The pain of the losers, but also their misguided decisions. Sometimes I am on both sides.

A few years into my teaching career, I was appointed Year Level Coordinator in a new school. The year after, I was entrusted with the responsibility to lead the oldest group in the school – year 11s. They were very rough around the edges and had not had a typical school experience. (Although, who has?) It was important to me that our once a week 'Pastoral Care' lesson was going to help them be the best they could be. It was obvious to me that they needed this – more than any students I had ever taught before.

Like many teenagers, they were at times brilliant, respectful, kind and capable – and at other times (too many times for many of them) they were apathetic, disinterested, lacking focus and unmotivated. Being a new school, we had not had a group of year 11s before (or a year 11 wellbeing program), so I began hunting around for schools that had – that part wasn't hard.

Then I arranged meetings with them – public schools, grammar schools, Catholic schools – to determine what they did best in their wellbeing programs. I found that they all had something to offer their students. However, despite the age of the school or the experience of the person looking after the program, they were still grappling. (By the way, I think this is a great thing – if we stop grappling, we stop learning.)

But it was more than that – they felt that what they were doing was not quite meeting the needs of the students. It was maybe not totally engaging, maybe a little outdated, maybe some of the messages missed the mark a little, and many of the teachers delivering it didn't seem to care too much for it. But they mostly persisted with it because they didn't have a great deal of time to create anything different and it seemed to be good enough to fill the slot.

I appreciated their honesty, their guidance and their willingness to share what they could to help someone starting a program from scratch.

But it caught my attention. In fact, it annoyed me a little. I got a little bee in my bonnet that has not since gone away. I was committed to improving what we shared with students. I could see that there was a huge need.

For me, I've always thought that equipping kids with skills to help them in their life, was just as important as helping them in their learning. I thought "If we don't teach our students how to set goals, maintain focus, persist, manage their wellbeing, communicate with each other, live with integrity, ride challenges, contribute positively to the world and influence others through their actions – who will?"

Kids need skills that will serve them well in their lives at school and beyond. If we want people to thrive, surely we should be teaching them some things that will help them be the best they can be- not just on the sporting field or in the classroom- as human beings. The curriculum is crowded and I would hate for such important things to be crowded out.

I was committed to changing the way staff thought about it too. But I didn't really have any ammunition.

Over the next three years I continued to meet with people in different schools and develop material in this space in order to benefit the students with whom I worked at my school. I took on the role of Assistant Principal within my school and sought to improve what we could offer our students in the area of Pastoral Care and Leadership (as well as a few other things, of course- but these areas were my passion). Part of my role was to mentor the school captains and student leadership team. In these meetings with high performing students in our school, I found that it was often the same issues that kept arising: attaching actions to their goals, setting priorities, forming good habits, managing their busy schedules, taking care of their wellbeing and managing stress.

At the other end of the spectrum, I was helping the least engaged and compliant students in the school as they struggled to take responsibility for their actions, stick to their learning targets, keep small commitments and look for continuous improvements.

The School Counsellors would tell me that many other students who came to them were struggling with stress, anxiety and depression. Often times, these were as a result of family or personal circumstances that were very painful.

I began to ask, "How can our students make better choices, if they don't have the skills? What options do they think they have? How can we as educators, be even more proactive? But honestly, who has time for that when there's so much work to be done right now?"

The bee was still in my bonnet.

As I read a little deeper into the research and findings of psychology, neuroscience and educational literature, I came across some research that I found interesting. I kept reading more on these topics and I was actually really surprised, at first. This stuff that I thought was so important and helpful to students, actually has a pile of evidence supporting it. Sure, not everything works, and not every topic needs three peer-reviewed journal articles to tell us what we know as professionals, but I was blown away by what literature was already out there. I was surprised that what I had experienced anecdotally in classrooms, playgrounds, parent teacher meetings and staff rooms, had been studied by researchers for their whole working lives.

This was fuel for the fire. After that, I was committed to helping schools grow in this area: building growth mindsets, building grit, building wellbeing and building leadership. Helping people live, learn and lead better. This has since become the focus of our work at UPP.

In 2015, I took leave from my job to see if my passion was something that would resonate with students and teachers in other schools. Over time, it seems that many educators in schools have begun to realise the importance of building growth mindsets, building grit, building wellbeing and building leadership for their students. Many people seem to want to improve in this area and offer their students the best material they can. Our vision is to help every student become their best. We aim to help students learn, live and lead better. As we continue to grow, our dream is now to impact 50,000 students every year through our exceptional incursions.

It's an exciting time to be working with schools in this area.

After all, in the words of Nelson Mandela, "Education is the most powerful weapon which you can use to change the world."

The world is changing at an increasingly rapid pace and students (as well as adults) need resilience as much as they have at any other time. Work intensification and the rise of technology have created an even greater need for a focus on wellbeing than ever before. And the concept of having leaders who are filled with integrity, committed to service and aren't just hungry for money or power is so important as our world moves into unknown territory.

So let's begin our journey together…

HOW TO USE THIS BOOK

Part 1 – Learning about Wellbeing and the elements of PERMAH
Part 1 of this book will focus on building a solid understanding of Wellbeing and PERMAH for those wanting to expand their knowledge and lead a Wellbeing / Positive Education initiative in their school context.

Part 1 is aimed at those people in school leadership teams or in middle level leadership positions who have a role in Pastoral Care/ Wellbeing/Positive Education in their school. A solid understanding of the topics taught to other staff and students would be helpful for those who are leading the charge in their own school context. Encouraging other key people on your work teams to read Part 1 may also increase their understanding and support of the initiative.

It has been divided into eight main sections, to make it easy for educators / readers to follow their own interest, and also to refer back to at a later stage, without having to read it from cover to cover.

It should be noted that Part 1 is not necessary for teachers of Pastoral Care/Wellbeing/Positive Education or individuals who are looking to apply the practices (although it may be helpful). If you are simply interested in doing the practices to improve your wellbeing or that of your students, you may prefer to skip Part 1.

Part 2 – Making Wellbeing Practical

While Part 1 will give people a greater understanding of the field, it is Part 2 that is focused on implementation and action. Part 2 will help educators and individuals to take the next steps forward in applying what you have already learned. For teachers of Pastoral Care/Wellbeing/Positive Education and those individuals who want to apply the practices, Part 2 will be more relevant and practical. The aim for Part 2 is to make wellbeing practical and give educators and individuals the tools to apply the findings of Positive Psychology.

Enjoy!

PART 1

Section 1 – An overview of wellbeing for schools

We all want to THRIVE! It's my fundamental belief that we all want to lead happy, healthy, engaged, purposeful lives. I believe we want to be connected to other people, to learn and grow, to prosper and to do good in the world. And yet, most of us struggle with this quest at one time or other in our lives.

More than a decade ago, I became a teacher so that I could help young people live the best life they were capable of living. I wanted to help every student become their best. I wanted to help school communities make even more of a positive impact on the young people who walked through their gates each day. I wanted to help those young people to function at a higher level so that their lives would be improved – for their own benefit and for the people around them.

My goal was not to help people avoid suffering. Instead, I became a teacher to enhance THRIVING. Since beginning this journey, I have become increasingly aware of the varied needs of young people. Some are really struggling, while some are thriving. As a result, I have looked to the research from positive psychology to determine what is helpful for those who are already doing well, as well as what may be helpful to those who are struggling. At different times during their life, an individual could well fall into both of those categories (as well as somewhere in between).

This study of positive psychology is aligned with my vision for education and the potential of each individual to live their best life. (Note that the tendency for us to sometimes think of our best life in competition with others, is ironically, not what I mean by our best life. In contrast, our best life is a life lived for others, or at least with others).

Positive psychology brings the rigour of the field of traditional psychology; however, it has a different focus and asks different questions. I believe that positive psychology, when applied, has tools that may be helpful to all of us (wherever we fall along the wellbeing continuum).

There are a few key themes that run through this book:

- We need to do the work to reap the benefits
  When it comes to wellbeing and positive psychology, learning about it is very different (and produces very different results) to actually doing it. We need to **'take the medicine' of positive psychology by actually doing the practices.** The Geelong Grammar model for Positive Education outlines that we should live it, teach it and embed it. Note that after we have learned something, it is the 'living it' that comes first.

  Just like a garden needs to be taken care of, we need to look after the soil, plant seeds, water the plants and tend to the weeds. In the same way, **we need to look after our minds like a keen gardener.**

  None of the strategies shared in this book will work if we don't actually do the work. There is no quick fix – it is about building positive habits that enhance our wellbeing.

- Prevention is better than cure
  Improving protective factors helps strengthen wellbeing and reduce the likelihood of poor mental health occurring. Additionally, being aware of mental health and wellbeing issues in ourselves and others helps us

to identify small issues and to get help for them before they become major issues.

- Mental health is a continuum
It's not as easy as thinking whether our mental health is good or bad. No matter who we are, mental health and wellbeing can be improved. We can all benefit from the practices outlined in this book. I encourage you to be proactive and build up your skills and resources in this area, regardless of how you feel right now.

- We need a range of tools
Maslow once said, **"If all you have is a hammer, everything looks like a nail."** Instead of young people only having one strategy when things are difficult, we would rather equip them with a range of tools that may be helpful. Then, they are better equipped for the ever changing landscape that lies ahead of them. **This book is a toolkit** that we can all draw on throughout our lives.

- It is far easier to pull someone down, than it is to push someone up
The law of gravity acts upon our bodies, and in a similar way, there are negative forces that can act on our wellbeing. It might be negative words, negative news, distraction, temptations and our fear of missing out (FOMO). This book aims to build human capacity in such a way that it will help people pull themselves (and others) up. We want people to flourish, and this is no easy task.

This book is countercultural:
I am fortunate to work on the **proactive side of the education system.** There does seem to be much toxicity in the world.

There seems to be a need for this work in our workplaces, families, hospitals, nursing homes, building sites and corporate environments. However, like most educators, my passion lies in empowering school communities, educators and students. This book is countercultural because it seeks to **build on the good things** in people's lives, and in school communities. To identify these good things and to magnify them.

This book is a work in progress:

The work of UPP is constantly evolving and improving, so this book could probably never be complete to the level that is required to do the messages justice. However, it seeks to help people, and it's clear that there is a great need. It seeks to make the world a better place. This book and the work that we do at UPP are our contribution to changing the world for the better ... fingers crossed!

Overview of wellbeing research

"Happy, calm students learn best." – Daniel Goleman

"Mental health is a state of wellbeing in which the individual realises his or her own abilities, can cope with the normal stresses of life, can work productively, and is able to make a contribution to his or her community." – World Health Organisation, 2004

"Health is a state of complete physical, mental and social wellbeing and not merely the absence of disease or infirmity." – World Health Organisation, 1948

Mental health is a positive and productive state of mind that allows an individual to respond to the challenges of everyday life. When we have positive mental health, we are more likely to enjoy relationships, benefit from opportunities and contribute productively to society. However, mental health cannot be taken as a given.

We are all vulnerable to changes in mental health, whether relatively minor and temporary, or more significant in duration and impact (Mind matters n.d.). We are encouraged to take action in order to restore, preserve and enhance our wellbeing. Much like we water the garden and pull out the weeds, we can also actively take care of our personal wellbeing.

Positive mental health and wellbeing are important for young people's ability to enjoy life, cope with the challenges they face, learn, engage with peers and adults and be well prepared for the future. Mentally healthy students tend to arrive at school ready to engage in learning and school activities and are more likely to achieve success (Mind matters n.d.).

The current state of play
Recent and emerging research indicates that our wellbeing is an area of need. This need seems to transcend culture, race, socio-economic status and religion.

Below is a glance at a few of the indicators:
- Depression rates today are nearly ten times higher than they were 50 years ago.
- The mean onset age of depression has sunk from 29.5 years to 14.5 years during this period (Seligman 2002).
- A 2004 study of Harvard students found that four out of five suffered from depression at one stage in the academic year, while nearly half of them were so depressed that it impacted their normal functioning (Kaplan 2004).
- It is predicted that by 2030, depression will be a leading cause of death, globally (Mathers & Loncar 2006).
- One in five Australians experience a mental health condition in any given year and almost one in two will experience a mental health condition at some point in their lifetime (ABS 2008).

- Nearly three million Australians live with depression and/or anxiety, which affect their wellbeing, personal relationships, career and productivity (ABS 2008).
- Only 35% of Australians with anxiety and depression access treatment (ABS 2008).
- Men are less likely to seek help than women, with only one in four men who experience anxiety or depression accessing treatment (ABS 2008).

Whether we like it or not, wellbeing is somewhat countercultural. Schools and workplaces are not typically overflowing with people who are thriving in terms of their wellbeing – and this has a cost on academic achievement in education and worker productivity in the corporate world. But all of that is really a conversation about disease, not wellbeing. So let's start the conversation about wellbeing with a focus on schools.

Why focus on schools?
If you wanted to improve the mental health of a nation, then a great place to begin is in schools. Almost everyone goes to school and in many communities schools are a central social hub. The impact of positive mental health action in school can extend well beyond the students' school life (Mind matters n.d.).

Adolescence (10–19 years) is a unique and formative time. Whilst most adolescents have good mental health, multiple physical, emotional and social changes, including exposure to poverty, abuse or violence, can make adolescents vulnerable to mental health problems. Promoting psychological wellbeing and protecting adolescents from adverse experiences and risk factors which may impact their potential to thrive are not only critical for their wellbeing during adolescence, but also for their physical and mental health in adulthood (WHO 2018b).

In particular, for adolescents:

- Suicide is the leading cause of death in Australia for 15-34-year-olds (ABS 2013).
- Long-standing research suggests one in five adolescents experience depression by the time they reach 18 years of age (AIHW 2011).
- Over 75% of mental health problems occur before the age of 25 (Kessler et al 2005).
- Focus on younger people is important, as research suggests that 50% of mental health conditions emerge by age 14, so it's vital to intervene as early as possible (Kessler et al 2005).
- Half of all mental health conditions in adulthood begin before the age of 14 (Lawrence et al 2015).
- Young people are less likely than any other age group to seek professional help (Slade et al 2009).
- Research shows that four out of five Australian teenagers think people their age may not seek support for depression or anxiety because they're afraid of what others will think of them (MediaCom Melbourne 2015).

Benefits of wellbeing practices in schools

Positive mental health strategies can help all staff, parents and students develop a greater sense of connection and belonging, as well as an increased sense of control, confidence and self-efficacy. Also, by promoting positive mental health and taking action when small issues appear we can help prevent the development of more serious mental health issues (Mind matters n.d.). Indeed, prevention is better than a cure.

While some educators believe that a focus on wellbeing takes time and resources away from academic pursuits, schools are increasingly becoming aware of the evidence that "students who thrive and flourish demonstrate stronger academic performance" (Norrish,

Robinson & Williams 2013). Students with high wellbeing gain higher grades and lower rates of absence (Suldo, Thalji & Ferron 2011), as well as higher self-control and lower procrastination (Howell 2009) and more creative, open-minded thinking (Fredrickson & Branigan 2005). Furthermore, positive mental health has been linked to increased enrolment, better retention of students, a positive school culture, and reduced behaviour management issues.

Based on this research, it is easy to see why wellbeing is an essential ingredient to thriving at school and beyond. Wellbeing for schools is not just about looking after our staff and students by helping them gain more peace, joy and happiness in their lives, although these are important. Wellbeing training for schools equips people with the skills they need to achieve more every day and also improves performance outcomes for our staff and students.

Indeed, wellbeing is a complementary goal, rather than a competing goal with academic performance. More and more schools seem to be prepared to embrace wellbeing practices and positive education. This research seems to support what many of the best educators have experienced anecdotally – with more than 90% of teachers agreeing that social-emotional learning is helpful for students (Bridgeland, Bruce & Hariharan 2013).

For many schools, wellbeing is the missing piece of the puzzle for developing their staff and students so they can take more productive and deliberate steps on their journey of thriving.

There are also many personal benefits of wellbeing practices.

Benefits to personal outcomes
Wellbeing is linked to success. It is related to our ability to function well in many areas. According to a meta-analysis involving

almost 300 studies and 275,000 people worldwide, wellbeing is linked to success in every domain in our lives, including marriage, friendship, careers, businesses, creativity and health (Lyubomirsky, King & Diener 2005).

Wellbeing is correlated with thriving in social, work, physical, psychological and personal domains. In one study, the wellbeing of employees was measured and these employees were followed for 18 months. Those who were happier at the start ended up receiving higher evaluations and more pay later on (Staw et al 1994).

In a different study of Catholic nuns, researchers found that those who were more overtly joyful in their journals at the age of 20 lived an average of 10 years longer than those who were more neutral or negative in their journals (Danner, Snowdon & Friesen 2001).

Finally, we look at the benefit at the organisational level.

Benefits to organisations

In 2002, a study was conducted to measure the levels of wellbeing for students starting university. This was found to correlate with their income levels 19 years later (Diener et al). Those with high levels of wellbeing also experienced higher job satisfaction and were less likely to have ever been unemployed. Employees with high wellbeing are more productive on the job.

Research has shown that those employees who are most unhappy take an extra 15 sick days off per year (Index 2008). Think of the cost to schools for relief teachers ... or the cost savings if each teacher could take one less sick day per year. Consider our students, who go to school 200 days a year for 13 years; 15 sick days per year would equate to an extra 195 days of school missed during their school career. This would put them a year behind their peers by the end of their years at school. Yikes! I still remember the one sick day I had in my five years of high school! How things have changed!

I have come across extreme cases where the absentee rate for particular students was more than 50 percent in a semester. This will have a very obvious impact on learning over the duration of a school career. And it would seem that these employees and students are not just taking 'sickies' or faking it.

Research shows that those with higher wellbeing experience higher resistance to the common cold. In one (slightly unethical) study, researchers measured people's emotional state and then injected them with a strain of the cold virus through nasal drops. A week later, the researchers found that those with higher levels of wellbeing were less affected by the virus. It wasn't just that they felt better. When measured by doctors, their physical symptoms – sneezing, coughing, congestion and inflammation were far less significant (Cohen et al 2003).

In Australia, businesses that spend money on employee mental health average a return of $2.30 for every dollar spent (PriceWaterhouseCoopers 2014). The direct financial impact on Australian business is in the vicinity of $11 billion every year, largely due to absenteeism ($4.7 billion) and reduced productivity ($6.1 billion) from unwell workers still attempting to work (Fells 2016).

This might be why "cutting-edge software companies have football tables in their employee lounge, why Yahoo! has an in-house massage parlour and why Google engineers are encouraged to bring their dogs to work" (Achor 2010). It also explains why many schools have embraced Wellbeing and Positive Education.

Risk and Protective Factors

Mental health can be broken down into three parts – risk factors, protective factors and resilience (Mind matters n.d.). This section will focus on risk and protective factors, while the next section will look at resilience.

Risk factors

"Risk factors are personal or social features that tend to be associated with poor mental health. When mental health is eroded by risk factors, then disruptive events may have an exaggerated impact and the person is at greater risk of mental health difficulties" (Mind matters n.d.). Risk factors will increase the chances of a negative health outcome occurring.

Some examples of risk factors are poor social skills, impulsivity, drug use, chronic illnesses or disabilities, family conflict or domestic violence, poor peer role models, exclusive school community, bullying/discrimination, racism, neighbourhood violence.

While the presence of one or more risk factors does not mean a student will develop a mental health difficulty, the more risk factors adolescents are exposed to, the greater the potential impact on their mental health (WHO 2018b). Through their ongoing contact with young people (and their families), schools may be in a position to reduce the impact of risk factors either by addressing a specific risk factor, or by strengthening protective factors. Many risk factors are outside a person's control. Therefore, it makes more sense to focus effort and attention on protective factors.

Protective factors

Protective factors tend to be associated with positive states of mental health. Protective factors tend to cushion and support us and minimise the effect of disruptions. They help to decrease the chances of a negative health outcome occurring.

Protective factors are conditions or attributes (skills, strengths, resources, supports or coping strategies) in individuals, families, communities or the larger society that help people deal more effectively with stressful events and mitigate risk in families and communities.

Examples of protective factors are physical health, good coping skills, social and emotional competence, connectedness and positive relationships, structure and support provided by family, clarity of values and behaviours, positive peer role models, safe environments, opportunities for achievement, participating in community networks, access to support services and a positive attitude to help seeking.

Protective factors reduce the likelihood of poor mental health. They may be thought of as assets that help people to maintain mental wellbeing and be resilient.

It is my opinion that wellbeing education in schools seeks to increase protective factors at the individual, peer and school level. For this reason, our work seeks to equip people with the tools and strategies they need in difficult times. Hence, our Personal Wellbeing Practices (PWPs) are a wellbeing toolkit for all members of the school community – but more on this later.

Mental health is shaped by risk and protective factors. However, the presence of these factors does not guarantee any specific outcome. A person with a large number of protective factors and no risk factors might still have poor mental health, while another person who seemingly has all the odds stacked against them might have very robust mental health.

The mental health continuum

Mental health is not fixed or static; it can change depending on our circumstances. Imagine a continuum with positive mental health at one end, emerging health difficulties in the middle and more serious mental health disorders at the other end. Depending on circumstances, an individual can move back and forth along this continuum (shown below).

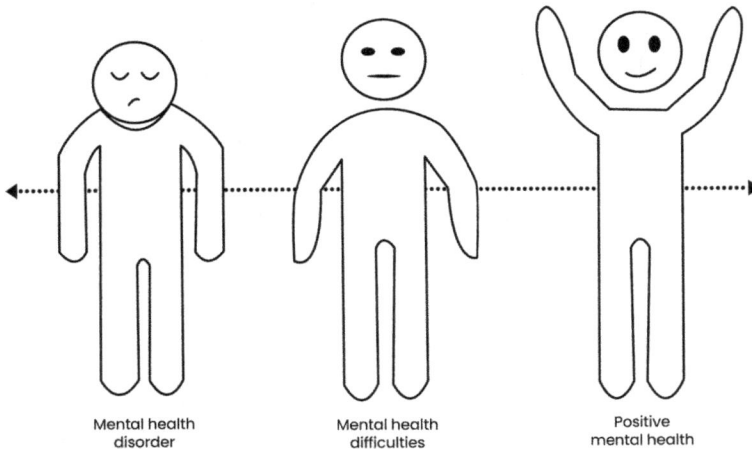

Mental health
disorder

Mental health
difficulties

Positive
mental health

Anyone can have a mental health difficulty at any time. These are not personality traits; they are experiences that many of us have. Sometimes we can resolve these difficulties by ourselves, and sometimes we could use extra support.

For people interested in learning more about this, you might like to check out Corey Keyes' dual continuum model for mental health and mental illness (the complete state model of mental health).

Prevention is better than a cure (intervention)

The best mental health strategy is the one that prevents issues from arising in the first place. So instead of being reactive and waiting for problems to arise, we can instead focus on promoting positive mental health. We may do this by creating a positive school environment and building strong relationships and connections throughout our school community. Then we can use strategies to develop resilience, particularly through equipping all members in our community with a toolkit of evidence-based practices that they can use in their own lives.

Of course, there are times when intervention is necessary and schools should certainly be supported by policies, procedures, referral processes, and internal and external support for those who are struggling with mental health difficulties.

Resilience Plus (+)

Resilience

Resilience is our ability to respond to disruptive life events and stressors. Our resilience is largely determined by personal skills such as emotional self-regulation and our social connections (Mind matters n.d.). It can be defined as: "The capacity to recover quickly from difficulties; toughness; the ability of a substance or object to spring back into shape; elasticity." (Oxford Dictionary 2018). Functioning well in our lives involves the ability to overcome difficulties, to take risks and to connect to other people.

Psychological resilience is the ability to successfully cope with a crisis and to return to pre-crisis status quickly (de Terte & Stephens 2014). Resilience exists when the person uses "mental processes and behaviours in protecting themself from the potential negative effects of stressors" (Robertson et al 2015). It allows us to remain calm during crises/chaos and to move on from the incident without long-term negative consequences. As humans, we utilise this evolutionary advantage to manage normal stressors in our lives. Those who possess resilience are likely to develop faster and be happier than those who bounce back from adversity more slowly.

Resilience allows us to cope with and adapt to new situations. Having a sense of resilience and positive wellbeing enables a person to approach other people and situations with confidence and optimism, which is especially important for young people given the enormous changes that occur with the transition into adolescence and adulthood (Reachout 2018).

However, is it possible to do more than just spring back into shape? Is it possible to positively adapt through certain disruptions in our lives?

Taking it a step further- Resilience Plus (+)
Resilience Plus recognises that there are times when we rebound from adversity as a strengthened and more resourceful person. The difficulty actually strengthens us.

Resilience is a process of positive adaptation that is developed as we "experience small exposures to adversity or some sort of age appropriate challenges" (Yates, Egeland & Sroufe 2003). I call this process of adaptive change and growth in our lives "resilience plus"- reminding us that in some situations, rather than simply bounce back (to where we were), it may be possible to bounce forward, as we learn, adapt and become better.

A similar thing happens when we go to the gym. Our muscles fibers actually break a little. Then, when we recover, our muscles are able to adapt and become stronger than they were before. Vaccinations use the same logic- injecting a person with a mild strain of a disease in order to become immune from the disease. There may be some merit in the saying- "what doesn't kill us makes us stronger".

Researchers use the term "post traumatic growth", to describe the transformation that can occur in people's lives after traumatic events. These events can lead to positive adjustments in our perspective, attitude and behaviours (Tedeshi & Calhoun 2004).

Resilience plus is different to post traumatic growth, in that resilience plus refers to bouncing back from small to medium difficulties that are inevitable in our lives, rather than life altering circumstances. However, I suggest that a similar process of positive adaptation can occur through the moderately difficult times of our lives.

So it may be quite helpful for our kids to lose at pass the parcel or musical chairs – not everyone wins a prize in all aspects of life. Michael Jordan famously said "I've failed over and over again in my life- and that is why I've succeeded." It's not that he succeeded despite lots of failure- he's succeeded because of it- because of what he learned from it, because he changed as a result. He didn't just put it behind him and forget about it. He stood on top of it. That's resilience plus.

How can we help to cultivate resilience plus in the lives of our students?

The good old days and the modern world

Dr Tim Elmore shares some brilliant thoughts on this, in an article entitled "How adults reduce grit in kids".

He notices that, when our parents grew up:
- Life was slower, with less technology and on-demand conveniences.

- Life was harder, with more manual labour jobs and do-it-yourself lifestyles.
- Life was more boring, with fewer screens and activities to entertain you.
- Life was quieter, without social media pinging at you night and day.

While these realities may sound depressing, they actually nourished grit in people's lives. With less glitz, glamour, noise and clutter, people stuck with something longer, even when the novelty wore off. There wasn't an expectation to be entertained; that everything would be fun or fast; or that that someone else would do the work we had been assigned.

Today's culture of speed and convenience frequently has led to a "Google Reflex", where we assume we can click and find answers in seconds. We don't have to memorize as much. We don't have to wait as much. We don't have to work as hard as we once did. We don't have to search as long.

But I'd like to focus here on the considerations for educators with big hearts who do want to help students be prepared for the inevitable challenges in their lives.

Considerations for educators

1. The more we do for them, the less they learn to do for themselves.
2. The easier life is for them, the less able they are to cope when challenges arise.
3. The faster their solutions come, the less they tend to take time searching for answers.
4. The more resources we give them, the less resourceful they become.

Helping by not helping

Resilience is not a trait that some people simply possess and others do not. There is no such thing as an 'invulnerable child' who can overcome any setback that they encounter in life. However, resilience is quite common. Masten (2001) refers to the "ordinariness of resilience," explaining that resilience is made of ordinary, rather than extraordinary, processes. This offers a more positive outlook on human development and adaptation. In particular, it overturns assumptions that children growing up with adversity will be worse off. That's not necessarily the case.

I think it helps if our kids don't have to learn these lessons later in life with the bigger things. (If they think everyone wins a prize in pass the parcel, how will they cope when they don't pass the test? How will they cope when they don't get the job? When they get dumped? When they miss out on their driver's licence?)

Parents and teachers are helpers – we want to help our kids. But sometimes that gets in the way of our kids being able to experience the "small exposures to adversity" that they need. The ideas of lawn mower parenting and helicopter parenting are well known. I think even as teachers, we should reflect on our willingness to "swoop in" to help and should instead consider allowing small mistakes, adversity and setbacks for kids. Resilience is, after all a dynamic two-way process between a person and their environment. We should consider "helping by not helping."

I have a confession to make – I, like many of you, admit to being both a parent and a teacher, so I am as guilty as anyone in this regard – I love to help. Although I have noticed that when I am able to sit back and watch a student (or our own kids) struggle to find the path (and then work it out), it is quite rewarding. Furthermore, this has been found to give children a sense of personal pride and self-worth (Steven & Wolin 2010).

Keep in mind that the adversity should be developmentally appropriate, as children do better when not exposed to high levels of risk or adversity. So if they can struggle and meet the challenge, great – help by not helping. But don't stand back while kids struggle with no pathway forward.

The point is that because many young people seem fragile and ready to give up at the first sign of setback, we tend to rescue them. As well as helping those in their time of greatest need, I suggest we focus on proactively equipping all students with tools to ride out challenges and manage their wellbeing. We need to build resilience before the stressful events- like building immunity to a disease with a vaccination. That's why wellbeing practices are so important. So what skills do they need?

The ingredients of resilience

The American Psychological Association (2014) suggests '10 Ways to Build Resilience', which are:
1. to maintain good relationships with close family members, friends and others
2. to avoid seeing crises or stressful events as unbearable problems
3. to accept circumstances that cannot be changed
4. to develop realistic goals and move towards them
5. to take decisive actions in adverse situations
6. to look for opportunities of self-discovery after a struggle with loss
7. to develop self-confidence
8. to keep a long-term perspective and consider the stressful event in a broader context
9. to maintain a hopeful outlook, expecting good things and visualising what is wished
10. to take care of one's mind and body, exercising regularly, paying attention to one's own needs and feelings

Contrary to what we might think, resilient people don't go it alone when bad things happen – they talk to the people who care about them and ask for help. While some individuals may be more inclined to have more of the list of resilient behaviours and attitudes, everything on the list can be increased.

Most of these elements are targeted through the toolkit we provide through our incursions for students and also through the Personal Wellbeing Practices in Part 2 of this book.

Positive Psychology Explained and History

"Positive psychology is an umbrella term for work that investigates happiness, wellbeing, human strengths and flourishing." – Shelley Gable and Jonathan Haidt

"Positive psychology is founded on the belief that people want to lead meaningful and fulfilling lives, to cultivate what is best within themselves, and to enhance their experiences of love, work and play." – Martin Seligman

Positive psychology explained

Positive psychology is "the scientific study of what makes life most worth living" (Peterson 2008) or "the scientific study of positive human functioning and flourishing on multiple levels that include the biological, personal, relational, institutional, cultural and global dimensions of life" (Seligman & Csikszentmihalyi 2014).

The term 'positive psychology' dates back at least to 1954, when Maslow's first edition of 'Motivation and Personality' was published with a final chapter entitled 'Toward a Positive Psychology' (Maslow 1970). At that time, much of the psychological field was particularly focused on trying to get people from poor wellbeing to neutral, or trying to "fix" people. There have been indications that psychologists since the 1950s have been increasingly focused on the promotion of mental health rather than merely treating mental illness (Secker 1998; Hales 2010).

Psychology's change in focus

"Before the second world war, psychology had three tasks: to cure mental illness; to improve normal lives, and to identify and nurture high talent" (Boniwell 2012). However, after the second world war, it seems that the last two tasks got lost, and the field focused almost solely on the first task – curing mental illness (Seligman & Csikszentmihalyi 2014). Psychology essentially operated from a disease model, asking "What's wrong with you?" and "How do we fix it?" Instead, this shift towards positive psychology is more of a matter of asking "What works?" or "What's right with you?" A focus on moving people along the wellbeing continuum is represented by the diagram below.

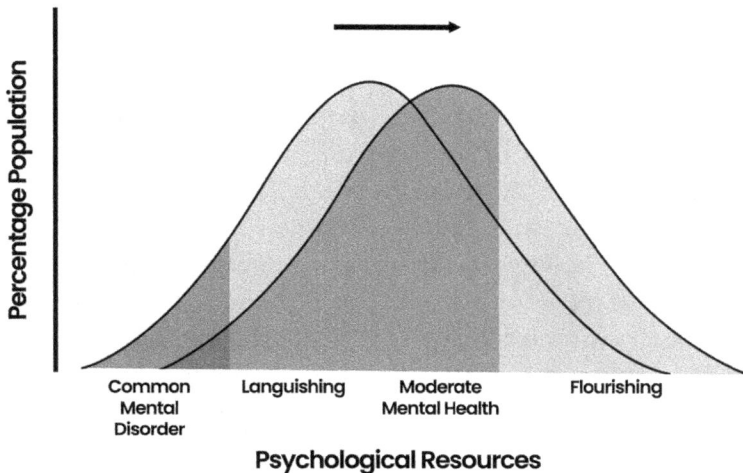

Moving the population towards flourishing (Huppert & So 2012).

Influences on Positive Psychology

Several humanistic psychologists, most notably Abraham Maslow, Carl Rogers and Erich Fromm, developed theories and practices related to human happiness and flourishing.

In 1984, Ed Diener published his tripartite model of subjective wellbeing, positing "three distinct but often related components of wellbeing: frequent positive affect, infrequent negative affect, and life satisfaction" (Tov & Deiner 2013).

Carol Ryff's six-factor model of psychological wellbeing (1989) postulates six factors which are key for wellbeing, namely: self-acceptance, personal growth, purpose in life, environmental mastery, autonomy and positive relations with others.

According to Corey Keyes, who collaborated with Carol Ryff and uses the term 'flourishing' as a central concept, mental wellbeing has three components, namely: hedonic (emotional pleasure), psychological and social wellbeing (Keyes 2002).

Positive psychology began as a new domain of psychology in 1998 when Martin Seligman chose it as the theme for his term as president of the American Psychological Association (Ben-Shahar 2007). He urged psychologists to continue the earlier missions of psychology of nurturing talent and improving normal life (Compton & Hoffman 2013). Seligman is a psychologist who became disinterested in studying different pathologies. He chooses to focus on exploring optimal human functioning – flourishing, rather than languishing. Mihaly Csikszentmihalyi, Christopher Peterson and Barbara Fredrickson are regarded as co-initiators of this development (Srinivasan 2015). It is a reaction against a focus on 'mental illness', which tends to focus on maladaptive behaviour and negative thinking. Instead, it encourages an emphasis on happiness, wellbeing and positivity, thus creating the foundation for what is now known as positive psychology (Srinivasan 2015).

Those who practise positive psychology utilise psychological interventions in order to build wellbeing (Seligman & Csikszentmihalyi 2014).

Positive Education

Martin Seligman defines positive education as "education for both traditional skills and for happiness." Positive Education seeks to combine the "implementation of scientific research and effective educational practice to enhance wellbeing, foster resilience and optimise engagement and performance" (Geelong Grammar School 2019). Wellbeing is not just about feeling good; it is not just the absence of pathology and illness. Instead, positive education focuses on taking people from wherever they are towards wellness.

While not all schools will value "positive education", as people may interpret that differently, at UPP we consider this to be synonymous with engaging, evidence-based wellbeing education and pastoral care. As a result, in this book, positive education is used interchangeably with wellbeing education.

This work has inspired my own passion and commitment for empowering people to live to their full potential. It's about thriving and continuously striving for personal excellence.

Research findings for Positive Psychology

A meta-analysis of 49 studies in 2009 showed that Positive Psychology Interventions (PPIs) produced improvements in wellbeing and lower depression levels. The PPIs studied included writing gratitude letters, learning optimistic thinking, replaying positive life experiences and socialising with others (Sin & Lyubomirsky 2009).

The results revealed that positive psychology interventions do indeed significantly enhance wellbeing. They also showed that we would do well to deliver positive psychology interventions for relatively longer periods of time – not just a one-off, but on a continuing basis.

In a later meta-analysis of 39 studies with 6,139 participants in 2012, the outcomes were positive. Three to six months after a PPI, the effects for wellbeing were still significant. However the positive effect was weaker than in the 2009 meta analysis; the authors concluded that this was because they only used higher quality studies. The PPIs they considered included counting blessings, kindness practices, making personal goals, showing gratitude and focusing on personal strengths (Bolier et al 2013). Many of these PPI's have formed the basis of our Personal Wellbeing Practices at UPP, although we have made them relevant for the school context.

This demonstrates that positive psychology interventions can be effective in the enhancement of subjective wellbeing and psychological wellbeing, as well as in helping to reduce depressive symptoms. Once again, the study demonstrated that effects were fairly sustainable over time and more effective if they were of longer duration.

Increasing self-efficacy

Self-efficacy is an individual's belief in his or her innate ability to achieve goals. Albert Bandura defines it as a personal judgement of "how well one can execute courses of action required to deal with prospective situations" (Bandura 1982). In personality psychology, locus of control is the degree to which people believe that they have control over the outcome of events in their lives, as opposed to external forces beyond their control. (Locus means 'location' or 'place' in Latin.)

Rotter (1996) states that our locus of control can be either internal (a belief that one's life can be controlled) or external (a belief that life is controlled by outside factors which they cannot influence). When we believe that we are able to benefit from the actions we take, we are more inclined to take them, and to reap the benefits. In fact, "there are no people who cannot benefit from applying positive mental health strategies" (Hassed 2008). The reality is that with the right tools, we all have the ability to improve our own wellbeing.

PERMAH – The Elements of Our Wellbeing

In 2011, Martin Seligman offered the PERMA framework in his book 'Flourish'. Many others have since added the H for Health. Each letter in the PERMAH framework refers to a pillar that contributes to our wellbeing, or what Seligman refers to as our level of 'flourishing'. Therefore, the six elements for our Wellbeing are: Positive emotion (P); Engagement (E); Relationships (R); Meaning (M); Accomplishment (A); and Health (H). Each of these can be developed, and the image below captures the six elements.

Positive emotion (P) encourages individuals to "anticipate, initiate, prolong and build positive emotional experiences" and accept and develop healthy responses to negative emotions (Norrish, Robinson & Williams 2013). Experiencing positive emotion has been found to benefit mental and physical health, social relationships and academic outcomes (Lyubomirsky, King & Diener 2005).

Engagement (E) involves living a life high in interest, curiosity and absorption and pursuing goals with determination and vitality (Norrish, Robinson & Williams 2013). Engagement is linked to wellbeing, learning and the accomplishment of important goals (Froh et al 2010; Hunter & Csikszentmihalyi 2003).

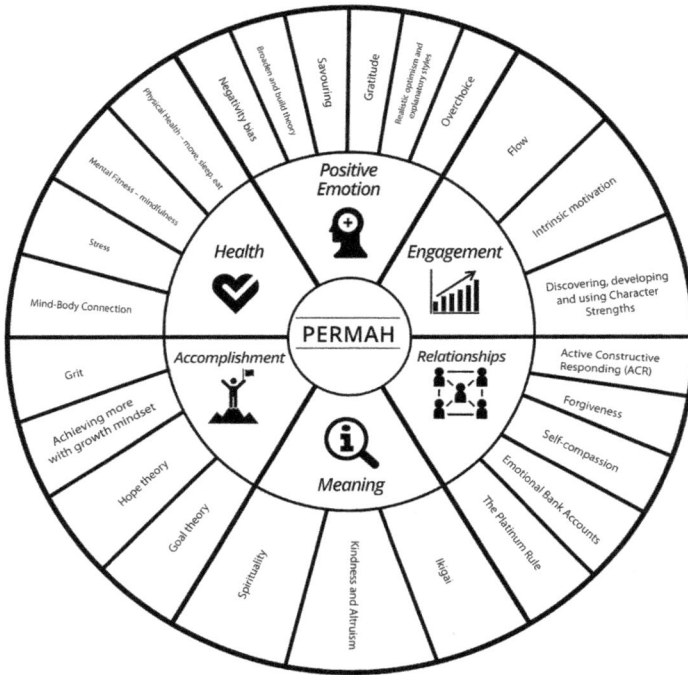

Relationships (R) consists of "developing social and emotional skills to enable the development of nourishing relationships with self and others" (Norrish, Robinson & Williams 2013). This is important because social isolation is a risk factor for depression, substance abuse, suicide and other symptoms of mental ill-health (Hassed 2008). On the other hand, supportive school relationships have been linked with child and adolescent wellbeing and resilience (Stewart et al 2004).

Meaning (M) is about developing an understanding of the benefits of serving a cause greater than ourselves and engaging in related activities (Norrish, Robinson & Williams 2013). Having a purpose in life is correlated to good physical health, high life satisfaction and strong relationships and is protective against depression and risky behaviours (Cotton Bronk et al 2009; Damon et al 2003).

Accomplishment (A) involves striving for and achieving meaningful outcomes (Norrish, Robinson & Williams 2013). Research suggests a bi-directional relationship between flourishing and positive accomplishment (Norrish, Robinson & Williams 2013). Mental health is a requisite for effective learning – it makes our minds available for learning (Hendren, Birrel Weisen & Orley 1994). In addition, the accomplishment of worthwhile goals leads to positive emotions and wellbeing (Sheldon et al 2010).

Health (H) refers to establishing habits that support positive physical and psychological health (Norrish, Robinson & Williams 2013). Research asserts that students who thrive physically and psychologically also perform well in their studies (WHO 2011). In addition, developing healthy behaviours in adolescence can carry benefits into later life, which reduces the risk of adverse health conditions such as diabetes or heart disease (Norrish, Robinson & Williams 2013).

The PERMAH model gives structure to Wellbeing and Positive Education. Without structure it is often difficult to set systematic, specific and achievable goals. Often it is good to work on one goal at a time, and as individual behaviours become established then move to the next goal according to motivation and priorities (Hassed 2008). Many of the aspects of PERMAH may benefit from the support and engagement of others such as family members and friends (Hassed 2008).

So, we now have a model for Wellbeing and Positive Education, but it has been my quest to determine the best way forward for schools. Since my studies with Dr Peggy Kern at the University of Melbourne, I have wanted to give schools a way to practise the research based Positive Psychology Interventions (PPIs). I feel like they are little pieces of gold, waiting to be discovered ... and that for many who have discovered them, it was difficult to know how the pieces fit together.

I figured that PERMAH provided an excellent framework. However, I wanted not simply to teach people about Wellbeing and Positive Education – I wanted more. I wanted to show people how to do some of the practices. I wanted to help them live it. I wanted something simple enough that students could do. And teachers needed to be able to model it, too. But it needed the rigour that this psychological science could provide. So, I needed to learn about the best method for delivery. Therefore, it was necessary to determine the characteristics of effective youth programs.

Characteristics of Effective Youth Programs

It is important to identify the characteristics of effective youth programs (Kern 2016), and consider these in light of any Wellbeing and Positive Education initiative in a school setting. These are outlined in the table below, along with the implications for what I was to develop.

It is understood that...	Implication for PPIs...
• Programs work best when guided by explicit theories.	• These materials will be organised based on the PERMAH framework.
• Longer-term programs are more effective than shorter intensive programs.	• The PPIs will allow for students to revisit the concepts/interventions at least each year.
• Active programs are most effective – especially those that develop skills through hands-on and minds – on engagement.	• There will always be immediate applications for the learners of PPIs, rather than just learning from a teacher, website or video. They will only include practical interventions that are directly applicable to school settings.
• The best programs are those in which youth have at least one supportive mentor.	• The PPIs will utilise the existing school structures that usually have students together with a (home room/pastoral care) teacher in the class for a period of one year (or longer).

(Adapted from Kern 2016)

Implementing Wellbeing and Positive Education in a Realistic Context

As an educator for many years before beginning the journey of Unleashing Personal Potential, I understood that there would be barriers to success in each school that attempted the journey of Wellbeing and Positive Education. I understood that this would include (among other things), inconsistency in delivery, lack of transferability to real life, lack of time and lack of a sequence for our PPIs. Each one of these barriers will be explained below, along with a brief explanation of how these barriers could be minimised.

Inconsistency of delivery

Inconsistency of delivery between classrooms within a school is the first likely barrier. Inconsistency could stem from variance in teacher knowledge and understanding of the content, variance in teacher ability to deliver on the PERMAH topics and also teacher 'buy-in'. These barriers could all be minimised (but realistically, not eliminated). One major way to minimise inconsistency is by investing time and professional development into the teaching staff to ensure they have had an opportunity to 'learn it and live it,' before being asked to 'teach it and embed it.'

Another way to minimise this inconsistency is to focus on one area each term, ensuring that staff are not overwhelmed by the demands placed on them. It has become clear to me through my studies and working with many schools that most schools that have had success implementing Wellbeing and Positive Education have demonstrated patience and perseverance in 'rolling it out' in their community. I would encourage schools to implement only what is manageable for them and not to rush the process. They should focus on quality of uptake by the community, rather than the number of things they can get their community to begin.

Transfer of skills and practices to real life

The second barrier is for students to actually be able to transfer the skills and practices they learn into their lives outside of school. One structure that might help students to do this is to expose students to these topics over the course of their time at school (not just in a short unit that they cover for a few weeks during one term).

The concepts should be revisited a few times during their school life, so that students continue to build their inventory or toolkit over time. This allows students to determine which are most helpful for them over time. Schools could also help students by 'embedding it' – by this, I refer to the idea of enculturating students with Wellbeing and Positive Education during their school life so that it is not seen just as something you do when you are in your wellbeing/Positive Education/Pastoral Care class. Rather, it should be seen as a set of skills and practices that can be referred to as the need arises.

Lack of time

Time will always be an issue for any initiative that is based in schools. It will take human resources to select, communicate and lead the implementation of Wellbeing and Positive Education initiatives and furthermore to assess the effectiveness in any school – and this is no small task.

My goal was to save people and schools time in resource development, so that they don't need to develop the material themselves (or read all the research, or study the courses). In fact, my work should be particularly helpful for those educators who have some understanding of Wellbeing and Positive Education, but lack the time to implement it. One way to turn this barrier into a strength was to ensure that whatever we developed was simple and easy to use.

Lack of sequence

The final barrier for schools is that it could be difficult for them to choose an appropriate direction or focus for starting Wellbeing and Positive Education. Schools may even have difficulty choosing a focus each week, fortnight, month or term. Some possible solutions to this could be allowing schools to choose whether they would prefer to focus on a particular focus area, or instead roll out a predetermined sequence that related to the needs of their school.

I also decided that it would be necessary to work closely with school personnel to help them develop a framework or direction that gives them focus. The beauty of having some tools for Wellbeing and Positive Education in the one place is that it would save schools a great deal of time and effort (because they don't need to find or create them 'in-house'). However, having them all in one place could still be very overwhelming. We want to steer clear of causing paralysis by analysis.

The fact that we can 'declutter' the wealth of material, research and information that exists and give schools practical steps is what they most value about the work we do at UPP. It may be necessary to provide the materials to schools in a default order (e.g. in the order of PERMAH) – not because that is the right order, but simply because it will take the difficulty in choosing away from them. Having said all of that, I think it is necessary for me to work closely with a few schools to ensure that we develop something that is very easy for them to navigate and use for this purpose.

Then I asked myself a big question:
How do we ensure we use an evidence-based model, apply what we know about schools, consider the characteristics of effective youth programs and give schools super practical tools that will help them on their journey of making wellbeing a reality?

My answer to this question was Personal Wellbeing Practices (PWPs).

Introducing Personal Wellbeing Practices by Unleashing Personal Potential

What is a PWP?

A Personal Wellbeing Practice (PWP) is an evidenced-based positive psychology intervention, applied in school communities or other educational settings. At UPP, as the creators of the PWPs, we have tried to make these PWPs simple, concise and relevant for students and their teachers. They include a rationale and an activity for teachers to implement with groups of students in less than 10 minutes each week. Each PWP will focus on one (or more) of the PERMAH elements.

Teaching and living the Personal Wellbeing Practices

An effective wellbeing program is not just a matter of knowing and understanding the different elements of wellbeing. In the same way that telling people about cardiac risk factors does not reduce cardiac risk (Syme & Balfour 1997), teaching people about PERMAH will not improve wellbeing. For wellbeing education to work, it must be practical. Rather than simply teach about wellbeing, we can support the information taught with strategies that empower individuals and improve 'control' or 'autonomy' (Syme 1998; Hassed 2008). This allows people to act on the information they have acquired and utilise the strategies that are helpful to them. This is why we have created the PWP's and is far more effective than simply learning about the six elements of PERMAH.

Wellbeing is something that changes over time. It is not static. Therefore, much like a garden that needs to be looked after (weeded, fertilised, watered, etc), we need to continue to cultivate the habits and practices that enhance our own wellbeing. Most of these activities can be revisited very regularly, require little or very

UPP's PERSONAL WELLBEING PRACTICES- LISTED BY TOPIC

POSITIVE EMOTION	ENGAGEMENT	RELATION SHIPS	MEANING	ACCOMPLISH MENT	HEALTH
One nice email (Staff PWP's)	Find a way to play (Staff PWP's)	Offer micro moves (Staff PWP's)	Volunteer yard duty (Staff PWP's)	Phone a friend (Staff PWP's)	Stop and eat lunch (Staff PWP's)
Broaden and Build Brainstorm- Wk 32	Strengths Reflection (Staff PWP's)	Do a 5 minute favour (Staff PWP's)	For the sake of what? (Staff PWP's)	Win the morning (Staff PWP's)	Leave the laptop (Staff PWP's)
Happy Memory Building- Wk 35	Stand up regularly (Staff PWP's)	Forgiveness- Wk 39	Get spiritual (Staff PWP's)	Turn off email alerts (Staff PWP's)	Mindfullness Strategies Wk 37
Overcoming Negativity Bias- Wk 33	Take a strengths pause (Staff PWP's)	Kindness Catching- Wk 38	Be awed by nature (Staff PWP's)	Best Possible Self and Dream Job- Wk 34	Mindful Walking- Wk 30
Sharing our grateful moments- Wk 28	Your Superhero Strengths- Wk 36	Active Constructive Responding- Wk 13	Awe Inspiring- Wk 25	A Gritty Person- Wk 17	3 Minute Stress Buster- Wk 29
Gratitude Letter- Wk 27	Savouring the moment- Week 31	Shout outs!- Wk 12 & Wk 40	Live your Legacy- Wk 24	Mindsets- Favourite mistake- Wk 15	Healthy Habits - Nutrition- Wk 21
Laugh out Loud- Wk 26	Intrinsic Motivation- Wk 16	Act of kindness- Wk 11	Make the mundane meaningful- Wk 23	Growth Mindset - Neuroplasticity- Wk 14	Healthy Habits - Sleep- Wk 20
Attitude of Gratitude- What went well- Wk7	Me at my best- Wk 10			Password Goals- Wk 4 & Wk 22	Let's get physical- Wk 19
Sharing hope- Wk 6	Flow activity- Wk 8			Goal Setting- T.O.P.- Wk 3	Staying Healthy- Wk 18
Happy Hits- Wk 5				3 hard things- Wk 2	Mindfulness body scan- Wk 9

few resources and only take a short time. They are all based on evidence that links them to increased wellbeing or other positive life outcomes. We will benefit from these aspects in our own lives. In addition, through modelling and teaching them, we pass them on and help our students, families and even ourselves to thrive.

The PWPs we have created aim to provide people with the tools to use to enhance their wellbeing. The following table provides a map of all of the Personal Wellbeing Practices on a single page.

Person Activity Fit

While each of the Personal Wellbeing Practices is supported by research in terms of having a positive effect, it is certainly not the case that 'one size fits all.' Not every practice works for everyone, all the time. Some people will find some practices more helpful than others. 'Different strokes for different folks' is also true for PWPs, meaning that some people will find certain activities more helpful to them personally, than other PWPs (Truempy 2014). This is known in the literature as 'person activity fit' (Sin & Lyubomirsky 2009).

The range of activities provided in this PWP inventory gives students and teachers access to a broad range of PWPs, over a long period of time at school. By offering students and teachers a buffet of PWPs to attempt, they will be equipped with a toolkit of strategies that they can choose to use to cope with the struggles and enjoy the highlights of life. It is hoped that people will use the PWPs that they find most effective and helpful for them in their daily lives, in order to move along the continuum of wellbeing towards flourishing.

Section 2 – Positive Emotions

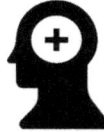

Positive Emotion

The Oxford Dictionary states that emotions are strong feelings deriving from one's circumstances, mood or relationships with others. However, this negates the fact that emotions can be caused by our own thinking patterns. Sternberg (1998) declares that an emotion is a "feeling comprising physiological and behavioral (and possibly cognitive) reactions to internal and external events."

Emotions actually produce change in physiology, thoughts and behaviour (Nairne 2000; Fredrickson & Branigan 2005). They are "nature's way of equipping us for the most fundamental task that faces us ... survival" (Gaffney 2011). Emotions affect "how we think, what we pay attention to, our relationships" and many aspects of our life (Lyubomirsky, King & Diener 2005).

A full range of emotions

It is most healthy to experience the full range of emotions. While feeling good involves living a life with frequent positive emotions, feeling good also involves giving oneself the permission to experience negative emotions without trying to deny or suppress them. The foundation of a happy life is not one with only positive emotions – it is one where we accept our full range of emotions and allow them to flow through us, without getting too attached (Ciarrochi et al 2013).

While there are many theorists who have developed different lists of emotions, Robert Plutchik's theory (1997) gives us a simple overview, explaining that the eight basic emotions are:
- Fear → feeling afraid, frightened, scared
- Anger → feeling angry, rage
- Sadness → feeling sad, sorrow, grief
- Joy → feeling happy, happiness, gladness
- Disgust → feeling something is wrong or nasty
- Surprise → being unprepared for something
- Trust → admiration is stronger; acceptance is weaker
- Anticipation → in the sense of looking forward positively to something which is going to happen. Expectation is more neutral. Excitement or nervousness would be two extensions of anticipation.

Pleasant and unpleasant emotions

Most of us would perceive some of the emotions as good/positive (trust, joy, anticipation) or bad/negative (anger, fear, disgust), although it may be more helpful to think of emotions as pleasant or unpleasant.

Unpleasant emotions are also valid and important. For example, one may feel sad (an unpleasant emotion) at the loss of a loved one, or we may feel angry when there has been an injustice served to ourselves or someone else. These unpleasant emotions would be helpful in that they will probably spark us into action. (We might seek support for ourselves and our grieving family, or we might stand up for what we believe in.) Fear may prevent us from doing stupid, unsafe things. Sometimes I wish my sons Elijah and Oscar had a little more of that healthy fear!

On the other hand, the abundance of pleasant emotions might not be helpful. Trusting too much (a pleasant emotion) may put us in harm's way. So pleasant or unpleasant emotions can be either helpful or harmful.

When we refer to positive emotion, we are referring to experiencing a full range of emotions in a healthy and helpful way.

Activating the prefrontal cortex with positive emotion
Richard Davidson has conducted research to determine which parts of the brain are involved in positive emotions. He found that the left prefrontal cortex is more activated when we are happy and is also associated with greater ability to recover from negative emotions as well as enhanced ability to suppress negative emotions. Davidson found that people can train themselves to increase activation in this area of their brains (Luz, Dun & Davidson 2007). It is now understood that our brain can change throughout our lives as a result of our experiences; this is known as neuroplasticity.

Negativity bias

Evolution has ensured that we feel the unpleasant emotions more strongly. This is called our negativity bias. The negativity bias is why "things of a more negative nature (e.g. unpleasant thoughts, emotions, feelings, interactions) tend to have a greater effect on our psychological state and processes than neutral or positive (pleasant) things" (Baumeister et al 2001). We tend to remember failures more than successes and analyse bad events more than good ones. Essentially, "bad is stronger than good" (Baumeister et al 2001).

Negativity bias in our daily lives
This effect is quite pronounced when we are driving our cars to work each day. Because people have such a strong aversion to loss, relative to gain, it often seems that the other lanes are going faster than the ones we are in. People on average change lanes every two kilometres. In one 1999 study by Redelmeier and Tibshirani,

120 people were shown a video tape of the traffic on a Canadian highway. Participants were looking through the eyes of a passenger in a car, which had a mounted video camera. Seventy percent of participants looked at the scene and thought the adjacent lane was moving faster, and 65 percent said in that situation they'd make a lane change. The reality was that the lane they were in was actually moving faster than the adjacent lane. But being overtaken hurts more than the joy of passing another car – this is due to our negativity bias.

Negativity bias is the human tendency to notice and be more influenced by unpleasant things and experiences, instead of more pleasant experiences. Examples of our negativity bias include remembering a bad day more easily than a good day, feeling like we are in the slow lane most often, or remembering insults instead of the nice things people say. Our brains react more strongly to negative input than positive input.

The origins of negativity bias – survival

We have a negativity bias because humans evolved to notice and respond more forcibly to the negative – this actually helped our ancestors stay alive. Negative emotions focus our energy on survival, which is fine if there is a lion in the classroom. While it is unlikely that a lion would be in the classroom, our brains are still wired to constantly be on the lookout for harm or danger. In most cases, this is unhelpful in our modern-day world. Left unchecked, the negativity bias can get in the way of our happiness and wellbeing.

Balancing the negativity bias

Knowing that we have a negativity bias can help us balance our negativity with positivity. While some negativity is necessary, or even helpful, our tendency to focus on the negative means that we need to outweigh the negativity in order to flourish.

Because our brains are like Velcro for negative (unpleasant) experiences and like Teflon (the stuff that makes frying pans non-stick) for positive (pleasant) ones, we need to intentionally notice and savour the positive experiences and feelings we have (Hanson 2010). We need three, four, five or six positive emotions to outweigh one negative emotion, although the exact ratio is hard to determine (Brown et al 2013) and will be different for everyone.

The value of higher positivity ratios

Within bounds, higher positivity ratios are predictive of flourishing mental health (Fredrickson 2013). However, it has been posed that when our positivity ratio reaches 11.5, flourishing begins to disintegrate and productivity and creativity decrease. They suggested as positivity increases, so too "appropriate negativity" (realistic feedback or constructive criticism) needs to increase (Fredrickson & Losada 2005). We should not live in a fairy tale world and endlessly seek only positive. However, by understanding that our experience of the negative will often outweigh the positive, it helps us to be aware that there will be times when we need to take proactive steps to increase positives. Ideas include scattering your day with things that you will enjoy, keeping a gratitude journal and savouring the good. But more on this in the PWPs section.

Broaden and build theory

As a result of our negativity bias, it might be easier for us to wallow in sadness, fear, anger or other negative emotions. However, this will lead to a narrowed focus, disconnection, lack of interest and less energy. Instead, we can develop skills to anticipate, initiate, experience, prolong and build positive emotions (Norrish, Robinson & Williams 2011). Doing so will help us to broaden our attention and build our skills (Fredrickson 2004).

Positive emotions broaden our outlook

While negative emotions tend to cause a narrow focus and restrict our attention, positive emotions cause broad, creative and flexible thinking and widen our attention (Fredrickson & Branigan 2005). Fredrickson (2009) says that "positivity opens us – it opens our hearts and our minds, making us more receptive and creative."

Positive emotions allow us to build our skills

This broadening of our attention tends to lead to being more willing to engage openly with the environment around us (whether it be people, nature, learning). This increased engagement with the environment leads to a building of physical, social, intellectual and psychological resources (Norrish, Robinson & Williams 2011). Fredrickson argues that "positivity transforms us for the better. By opening our hearts and minds, positive emotions allow us to discover and build new skills, new ties, new knowledge and new ways of being."

Positive emotions improve our physical health

Furthermore, an increase in positive emotions can lead to the release of hormones and neurotransmitters that have a protective and beneficial impact on our physical health and immune functioning (Pressman & Cohen 2005), in particular, serotonin and dopamine (more on this in Section 7.1, Mind-Body Connection). This occurs via the reduction of the stress response (fight or flight) and increasing the activity of the parasympathetic nervous system (rest and digest).

Frequency is more important than intensity

"Happiness or wellbeing, is more strongly associated with the frequency and duration of people's positive feelings, not with the intensity of those feelings" (Diener 2009). So it is well worth calling to mind some of the small positive occurrences in our lives, rather than waiting for our next 'theme park' experience. On a personal note, I would rather plan a couple of nice weekends away with the family each term, rather than planning one big holiday every two years. The regular weekends feel like it is part of my life, whereas the one big holiday feels like it's a holiday away from my life. This practice is really trying to build frequency rather than intensity.

Rather than grasping positive emotions too tightly, we are better off to increase the frequency of positive emotions through daily life (Fredrickson 2009). Think 'FOMO' (fear of missing out) – it's funny how we are so concerned with missing out on something big in our lives, when sometimes we don't even notice the sunrise, the sand between our toes, the smile of our child, the respect between two friends, the excellence of a colleague etc. In this way, I think our own 'FOMO' on the next theme park experience actually leads to us missing out on what we have right now.

Benjamin Franklin once famously said that "happiness consists more in small conveniences or pleasures that occur every day, than in great pieces of good fortune that happen but seldom." Jim Rohn (2017) puts it another way – "Wherever you are, be there."

A few ideas about positivity:
Positivity feels good, broadens minds, builds resources and fuels resilience. Ratios above 3:1 forecast flourishing. People can raise their positivity ratios.

Here are 12 tools/strategies to raise your personal positivity ratio from Barb Fredrickson's book, 'Positivity' (2009):
1. be open
2. create high quality connections
3. cultivate kindness
4. develop healthy distractions
5. dispute negative thinking
6. find nearby nature
7. learn and apply your strengths
8. meditate mindfully

9. meditate on loving kindness
10. ritualise gratitude
11. savour positivity
12. visualise your future

There are numerous strategies that we can use in order to enhance our positive emotions (and limit our negativity bias) in order to broaden our attention and build our skills. UPP incursions do this in a way that allows students to engage with many of these strategies, and so too do the PWP's we have included in Part 2 of this book. In particular, I will focus on savouring, gratitude and realistic optimism. These will be outlined in the rest of this section.

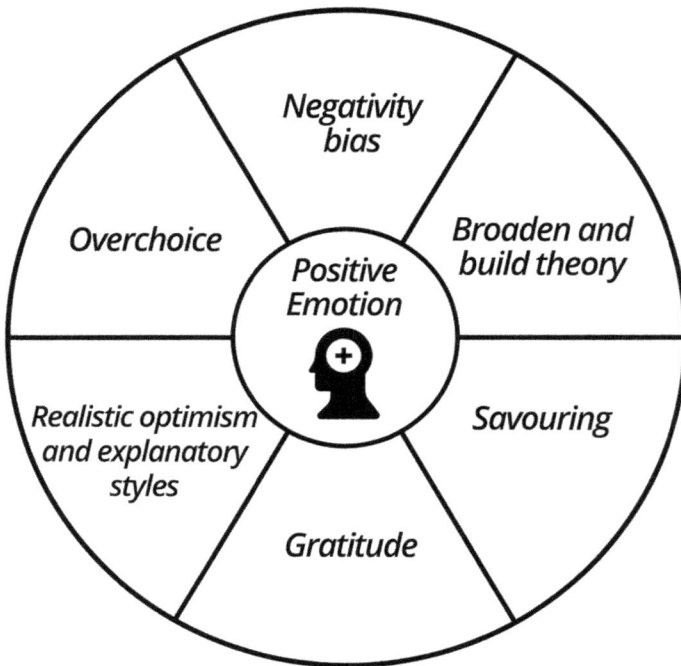

Savouring

To savour is to "enjoy or appreciate (something pleasant) to the full, especially by lingering over it" (Oxford Dictionary 2018). If you savour an experience, it is like swishing the experience around … in your mind (Bryant & Veroff 2006). It is possible to savour the past, present or future. We can savour the past by reminiscing, sharing previous experiences, or thinking about past success. Savouring in the present involves focusing our attention on the good things in the 'here and now' (like a delicious taste or smell, or a special moment shared with someone). Savouring the future involves planning for exciting events in the future.

To put this into practice, check out the relevant PWP (Week 31), in part 2 of this book.

Gratitude

"Gratitude is when memory is stored in the heart and not in the mind." – Lionel Hampton

"He is a wise man who does not grieve for the things which he has not, but rejoices for those which he has." – Epictetus

"Give thanks in all circumstances." 1 Thessalonians 5 (Biblica 2018).

Gratitude is the "quality of being thankful; readiness to show appreciation for and to return kindness" (Oxford Dictionary 2018). Gratitude is associated with good physical and mental health (Wood, Froh & Geraghty 2010); it increases positive emotions and it combats our negativity bias. Gratitude has been found to increase happiness by as much as 25% – and these increases are largely sustainable (Emmons 2007).

"By cultivating gratitude, we are free from envy over what we don't have or who we are not. It doesn't make life perfect, but with gratitude comes a realisation that right now, in this moment, we have enough, we are enough" (Emmons 2007). We might hope to "feel and express [true] gratitude frequently" (O'Connell et al 2017).

Research has underscored the importance of gratitude to psychological and physical wellbeing (Emmons & McCullough 2003). Students (aged 11 to 14) who wrote three good things each day reported more satisfaction and enhanced wellbeing levels, particularly those who were lower to start with (Froh et al 2007).

Priming our brain with gratitude

Few things in life are as integral to our wellbeing as gratitude. Gratitude trains our brains to scan our environment and focus on the positive. When we are looking for things to be grateful for, we tend to find them. Psychologists call this process of priming your brain to remain on the lookout for opportunities 'predictive encoding'. They have found that priming your brain to expect a favourable outcome actually encodes your brain to recognise the outcome when it arises (Siefert & Patalano 2001). It makes us about 3 times more likely to notice a positive. In the words of Henry David Thoreau, "It's not what you look at that matters – it's what you see."

People who choose to be grateful wire themselves for more joy, opportunity and positivity. So, it is worthwhile to be a 'glass-half-full' sort of person. It has been said that the glass is in fact always full – half full of water and half full of air…

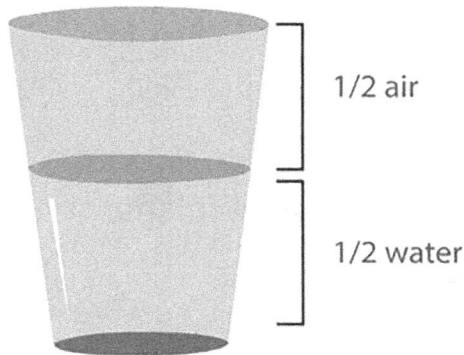

1/2 air

1/2 water

Technically,
The Glass is always Full

While religions and philosophies have long embraced gratitude as an essential ingredient to wellbeing and thriving, scientists have been late to recognise this concept. However, there is a growing body of evidence revealing the many benefits of gratitude.

Practising gratitude

Daily gratitude practice resulted in higher reported levels of positive states such as alertness, enthusiasm, determination, attentiveness and energy (Emmons, n.d.). In addition, gratitude correlates with goal attainment, high energy, positive moods, quality of sleep and more positive attitudes towards school and family (Emmons & McCullough 2003). However, Brene Brown at the University of Houston says that having an "attitude of gratitude" or simply "feeling grateful" isn't enough. Instead, we require tangible gratitude practices such as gratitude journals, gratitude jars, gratitude letters and family gratitude rituals (Brown 2012).

There are some simple practices that parents, educators and students can do to cultivate gratitude in our lives. Some of these include common gratitude exercises: gratitude visits; gratitude letters; what went well (aka three blessings or three good things); gratitude journals, creating a gratitude poster/book, gratitude present and gratitude 365 or 31 (recording gratitude for 365 or 31 days in a row).

Realistic optimism and explanatory styles

The importance of optimism

Optimism is "hopefulness and confidence about the future or the success of something" (Oxford Dictionary 2018). On the other hand, pessimism is "a tendency to see the worst aspect of things or believe that the worst will happen." Optimists (when compared to pessimists) tend to experience less distress in difficult moments or negative events in their lives, they tend to exert more continuous effort and tend not to give up easily, enjoy better physical health, engage in more health promoting behaviours (Boniwell 2012) and are more productive in the workplace (Carver & Scheier 2002).

The way that we can identify our own optimism or pessimism is through looking into our explanatory styles.

Explanatory styles

Explanatory style refers to the way in which we explain the causes and influences of previous events.

Ilona Boniwell writes in her book 'Positive Psychology in a Nutshell' (2012), that "a pessimistic explanatory style means we use internal, stable and global explanations for bad events, and external, unstable and specific explanations for good ones." People who use the pessimistic explanatory style tend to appraise bad events in terms of personal failure.

An optimistic explanatory style, on the other hand, is characterised by external (leaving one's self-esteem intact), unstable (temporary) and specific (depending on circumstances) explanations for bad events and by the opposite pattern for good ones."

A summary of this approach to explanatory styles is outlined here:

Personal	Is this situation related to internal or external causes?
Permanent	Is this situation stable (lasting) or unstable (temporary)?
Pervasive	Is this situation global (affecting many things) or local (specific to this situation)?

An example of the optimistic explanatory style
For example, an optimistic teacher who did not get the promotional position they applied for might think:

Personal: this is related to external causes	"The other applicants were excellent."
Permanent: this is temporary	"I will try again next year."
Pervasive: this is specific to the particular role	"Maybe I would have been more successful if this job was at a smaller school."

The downside of optimism
The above example is optimistic. The individual is able to protect themselves from self-loathing and it will help them to be at less risk of falling victim to negativity bias. However, it is not always best to be optimistic. For instance, optimism can lead to an underestimation of risks (Peterson & Park 2003), therefore optimists are more likely to take part in high-risk activities like

unprotected sex or reckless driving. Also, it may not be wise to be too optimistic about a situation involving personal health or an upcoming exam. ("She'll be right mate" may be optimistic, but not sensible.) In many cases, an optimist might remain naive to the realities and continue to live in their bubble – slightly detached from the reality of the situation.

Realistic optimism – a better alternative

Ed Diener writes that "It might not be desirable for an individual to be too optimistic" (2003). As a result, realistic optimism might be a better way forward for us. The key to success here is to monitor and recognise our thoughts. In particular, we are able to do this by monitoring and adapting our explanatory style.

Realistic optimism would likely be better than optimism in the example above regarding the teacher who missed out on a position they were hoping for. Realistic optimism might help the teacher to realise that they weren't quite ready for that role yet or that they need to learn more skills in a particular area before applying again. In some cases, the optimist and the realistic optimist might actually be in alignment in their thinking (e.g. it could be true that they are ready for the role and that they would be more successful in a smaller school). However, the realistic optimist has a slightly more healthy and objective perspective of the situation.

Learning realistic optimism

Learned realistic optimism contrasts with learned helplessness, which consists of a belief, or beliefs, that one has no control over what occurs, and that something external dictates outcomes such as success. Realistic optimism is learned by consciously challenging negative self talk. This includes self talk on any event viewed as a personal failure that permanently affects all areas of the person's life (Alarcon, Bowling & Khazon 2013).

Overchoice – becoming a 'satisficer'

We live in a time when we have the world at our fingertips. We have choices. So many TV channels, so many websites, so many types of cheese at the shop, different varieties of pet, many different leisure pursuits on offer. However, this is not always a great thing. We can get lost in the array of choices open to us. "The fact that some choice is good, doesn't necessarily mean that more choice is better" (Schwartz & Ward 2004). Oftentimes, we can feel a sense of overwhelm at the large number of decisions that require our attention and energy.

An overload of choices actually results in a rapid reduction of choices made. We tend to get 'paralysis by analysis'. In this case, we use all of our decision making power in so many little decisions – when, to be honest, there are more important things in the world than which type of paper I would like to print on this week. This "first-world" problem is called overchoice.

Satisficers and Maximisers

The best remedy for overchoice is to be a 'satisficer', rather than a 'maximiser'. A satisficer is a person who just needs to get what is good enough for their requirements. They consider options until they find what meets their minimum criteria and then they select that option. Maximisers are those who need to get absolutely the best deal and so look at all possible options.

Choice overload is a problem for maximisers who want to go to the best school, get the best job, have the best car and wear the best clothes. As more options become available, they need to work harder to exhaust all the possibilities" (Boniwell 2012). Maximisation is negatively associated with happiness, optimism, satisfaction with life and high self-esteem, while it is positively correlated with regret, perfectionism, depression and comparing ourselves with people who have more than us.

So what can we do about it?

Toffler (1970) offers some useful suggestions:

- 'Freeze-up' decision making when we are feeling overloaded (commit to not taking on anything new)
- Create 'stability zones' with long-term relationships and daily habits
- Defer or delay purchasing items that we don't need

Additionally, Barry Schwartz (2004) offers the following ideas in his book entitled 'The Paradox of Choice – Why more is less':

- Know when it is okay to accept 'good enough'
- Avoid social comparisons – set our own standards and don't try 'Keeping up with the Joneses' (which is increasingly difficult in the age of social media where most people show only the parts of their lives that they wish to share)
- Be grateful for what we have
- Learn to love our constraints (e.g. job, children, etc) because these things actually reduce the number of choices available to us
- Create rules for certain things in our lives so that we can limit our decision making energy

Doing these things helps us embrace the notion of being satisfied with our lives as they are now. We can increase our awareness of 'JOMO' (joy of missing out) and let go of 'FOMO' (fear of missing out). Doing so will aid us in building our positive emotions.

Subtraction and elimination are useful when it comes to tackling the problem of overchoice in our lives.

Subtraction for productivity

Many people find that they become more productive if they remove the things that conflict with their decisions or that make their decisions difficult. Life can be made easier if we delete whatever is unnecessary from our environment so that it makes it easier to stick to our decisions and helps us to develop good habits, rather than by forcing us to make decisions and exercise our willpower. Otherwise, our environment creates friction for us – by using up decision making energy in the very small aspects of each day.

For example, I am much more productive in my reading, writing and development of new materials when I close the emails tab on my computer. I am much more able to be present to my wife and children when I don't have my phone with me. This is subtraction for productivity.

Elimination is often the fastest way to progress and gain forward momentum. Many people find that 'less is more'. So, what things can you delete from your environment?

- ELIMINATE STUFF – clean out your wardrobe and your car, delete unused phone apps, clear out the pantry and fridge. The less stuff you have to clutter up your life, the fewer decisions you need to make each day.

- ELIMINATE DISTRACTIONS – Dopamine is a neuro-transmitter in the brain that is associated with pleasure. It's intended to help us make correct choices, but these days many of us are out of whack – checking email and social media, mindlessly surfing the web, eating something sugary and sweet – all of these activities release dopamine. Removing the distractions that give us these guilty pleasures allows us to concentrate on what is really important – whether that is being more productive at work or spending quality time with our family.

- ELIMINATE OPTIONS – Having more options is not necessarily a good thing. It can lead to indecision and half-committed choices, and we are left unsatisfied and wondering if we made the right choice. Sometimes, options serve as nothing more than distractions, so if we can eliminate some of those options it can help us remove some of the internal conflict from our life. The fewer choices we have to make, the more powerful our choices will be.

- ELIMINATE PEOPLE – Whilst having friends and colleagues is important, it is also important to choose your friends. Sometimes we need to actively cultivate our friendship groups so that we spend more time with those whose lifestyle and habits are most like our own (or like the habits we would like to have). As Dan Sullivan said, "Surround yourself with people who remind you more of your future than your past."

- ELIMINATE BRAIN CLUTTER – Our brains are wired so that they remember the important things – not every minor detail of our lives. Our head is built for having ideas, not for holding them. When you get a flash of insight or some new idea, immediately record it. Get it down on paper or record it in audio. Outsource your thinking to your environment to free your working memory space – e.g. get a journal, use a calendar you can write on, use quick voice on your phone, have a post-it note pad beside your bed.

Subtracting, eliminating and deleting is a genuine path forward to a slightly more simple life. I suggest you try just one of these strategies this week. If it makes a difference to your wellbeing, stick with it.

Practices to build Positive Emotions

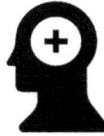

Positive Emotion

POSITIVE EMOTION	
One nice email	Set a reminder on your calendar to send one nice email to a colleague each week. This should be someone who has done something noteworthy or excellent.
Happy memory building	Think of a great, feel good memory that you shared with another person. Relive that memory in your mind. Next time you see the person, share the memory with them (or you could text, call or email them immediately). *PWP Wk 35
Overcoming negativity bias	Reflect on one negative experience that happened yesterday or today. Now think of some positive experiences and choose three to write down. Spend a moment savouring the positive emotions from the good things that happened. *PWP Wk 33

Broaden and build brainstorm	Think of something that makes you feel happy. It might be a place, a person, a great memory, a beautiful picture, your favourite music or meal. Spend a few moments with those happy thoughts. (You don't need to share these with anyone.) The goal here is simply to increase positive emotion so that you are more able to broaden and build. *PWP Wk 32
Sharing our grateful moments	Think about a moment in your life that you are grateful for. It can be big or small. Share this moment with a colleague or family member. Explain how it made you feel and why it happened. *PWP Wk 28
Gratitude letter	Think of a person who you would like to meaningfully thank because they have helped you, been kind to you or had a positive influence in your life. Write a short letter to this person expressing your appreciation for how they have impacted you. Share the letter with them. *PWP Wk 27

Laugh out loud	Research a few jokes (and share them with a friend). The challenge is to respond with wild laughing – real or fake – as the body doesn't know the difference. The fake laughing usually leads to real laughing anyway. *PWP Wk 26
Attitude of gratitude – what went well	Think about three things that went well in the past week (or day). They can be small, but should be things for which you feel grateful. Write down the three things that went well in your journal. *PWP Wk 7
Sharing hope	Spend a few moments thinking about one thing you are really looking forward to in the next month. With a friend or family member, take turns to share what you are looking forward to and why. *PWP Wk 6
Happy hits	Write down three happy thoughts – things that bring a smile to your face. For example: a favourite song, a great memory, a funny YouTube clip you've seen, a person who makes you smile, a place that brings you peace, a funny scene from a movie. Share these with someone you care about. *PWP Wk 5
* For more information and to lead this practice with your students, go to the relevant PWP in Part 2.	

Section 3 – Engagement

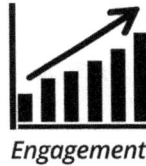

Engagement

To engage means to "occupy or attract (someone's interest or attention)" or to "establish a meaningful contact or connection with" someone or something (Oxford Dictionary 2018). Being engaged involves living with a high degree of interest, attention and connection. While disengaged individuals are bored, apathetic and alienated, engaged people are typically more curious, interested, motivated and persistent (Ryan & Deci 2000).

Engagement has been found to predict life satisfaction, gratitude and prosocial behaviours (Froh et al 2010) while it can reduce participation in at-risk behaviours (Nakamura & Csikszentmihalyi 2014). Research also suggests that the most interested and engaged adolescents tend to have an internal locus of control – that is, they feel as though they are mostly in control of their actions and circumstances (Hunter & Csikszentmihalyi 2003). As we look at the element of engagement, we are going to explore the topics of flow, intrinsic motivation and character strengths.

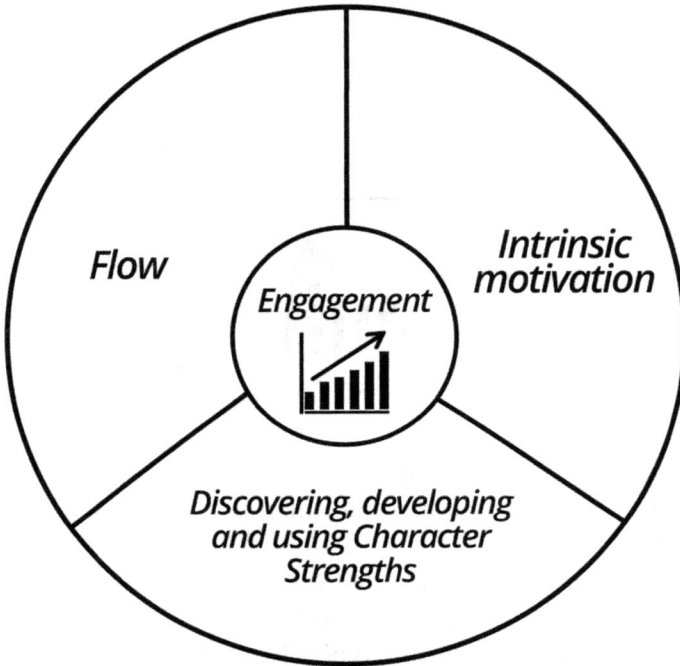

Flow

> *"Flow is the mental state of operation in which a person performing an activity is fully immersed in a feeling of energized focus, full involvement, and enjoyment in the process of the activity."* Mihaly Csikszentmihályi (2013).
>
> *"Flow is an optimal state of consciousness where we feel our best and perform our best. It is total absorption in a task and total focus."* Steven Kotler (2015).

Characteristics of flow

Have you ever lost track of time or been totally absorbed in a task? You may have been in a flow state, which is characterised by:

- Intense and focused concentration on the present moment
- Merging of action and awareness
- A loss of reflective self-consciousness
- A sense of personal control over the activity
- Losing track of time
- Experience of the activity as intrinsically rewarding (rewarding for its own sake – not particularly for an outcome) (Csikszentmihalyi 2013).

The neurochemistry of flow and the benefits for learning

A flow experience causes a cascade of neurochemicals – adrenaline, dopamine, endorphins, anandamide and oxytocin – to be released into our brain (Kotler 2015). This is the most potent concoction our brain can develop – a natural high. It makes us feel good.

Not only that, these experiences are performance enhancing. Creativity has been shown to increase 500-700% in a flow state. Military marksmen are 230% faster at shooting when they have been led into a flow state. The time taken for people to go from novice to mastery level in tasks such as archery has been cut in half. We tend to take in more information faster, link together related ideas more readily (allowing us to synthesise at a higher level) and also connect different ideas more readily (which improves our lateral thinking) (Kotler 2015).

Flow allows us to truly focus our energies on one thing, which results in much higher mental output. The neurochemical dump that is experienced during a flow state helps our brain to better tag our learning experiences. Steven Kotler asserts that it "jacks up learning." In particular, the more neurochemicals that show up during an experience, the more chance of moving the experience from short-term holding into long-term storage in our brain (Kotler 2015).

Flow increases concentration. Our nervous system can process about 110 bits of data every second. Seems like a lot. However, when we listen and seek to understand someone, that uses up about 60 bits of data per second (Csikszentmihalyi 2013). This is why we struggle to understand two people talking to us at once. (It is also part of the reason why talking on the phone while driving [even hands-free] is dangerous.) Our brain is only free to receive an extra 50 bits of data. If we are a less experienced driver, that may not be enough free 'brain space' to be proactive and safe on the road.

Flow has a documented correlation with high performance in the fields of artistic and scientific creativity, teaching, learning and sports. In addition, it has been linked to persistence and achievement in activities while also helping to lower anxiety during various activities and raise self-esteem (Nakamura & Csikszentmihályi 2014).

A word of warning about flow

It is also worth noting that flow does have a shadow side. Sometimes, high levels of curiosity and novelty (which are often associated with flow) lead to more risk taking behaviours (Schuler & Nakamura 2013). Sometimes our students might find flow playing computer games (Fortnite or Call of Duty). This does not happen by accident. Video game designers are aiming for optimal engagement and trying to provide the experience of flow for gamers. Just because we are in flow, does not mean that we are doing life-giving or adaptive activities.

Some of our flow may be counterproductive, and in this way, it could be quite addictive. Knowing that in some way as educators, we are competing with the rest of the world for the focused attention of our students, it might be helpful to understand how we can increase the likelihood of flow (for ourselves and our students) in helpful and useful ways.

What causes flow to happen in the classroom?
So what factors are conducive to flow and what can we do as educators to create these optimal learning conditions?

There are three main conditions that can lead to flow (Csikszentmihályi, Abuhamdeh & Nakamura 2005):

- Clear goals and purpose – It makes sense that we identify and articulate learning intentions and success criteria at the start of a lesson.
- Clear, immediate feedback – this does not always need to be from the teacher – it may be peer to peer, or most often, students would get feedback from their progress on the task at hand – although this is very difficult if they don't have a clear goal/purpose/learning intention to shoot for.
- A balance of challenge and skills – this emphasises the need for differentiation in our classrooms, as the aim is to match the challenge to the perceived skills, to ensure that each student is able to 'stretch' their skills. A slight stretch is best. High challenge and high skill is where we are most likely to find flow. (See diagram below for a simple illustration of this point.)

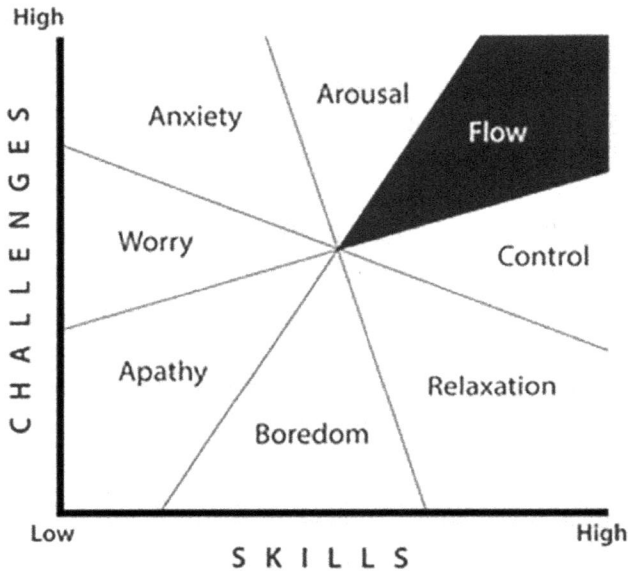

The likely experience as a relationship between challenge and skill (Kahn 2003).

When skills are high and challenges are low, for example, a person can experience states like relaxation or even boredom; when challenges are high and skills are low, anxiety or worry can result; when both skills and challenges are low, a person can experience apathy. When challenges and skills are matched at a high level, the resulting state is flow (Kahn 2003).

> *"The best moments in our lives are not the passive, receptive relaxing times. The best moments usually occur if a person's body or mind is stretched to its limits in a voluntary effort to accomplish something difficult and worthwhile."* Mihaly Csikszentmihalyi

Teachers can't control everything, but …

Let's be clear – teachers cannot create a flow state within their students. However, they can create environments where the flow state is more likely to occur by providing clear goals, feedback and challenges that match participants' perceived skills. When they get students in their flow state, the neurochemical bomb that is created could lead to higher outcomes. One other consideration – flow is highly contagious. So flow environments could be key to high quality learning environments.

Intrinsic motivation

> *"Perhaps no single phenomenon reflects the positive potential of human nature as much as intrinsic motivation, the inherent tendency to seek out novelty and challenges, to extend and exercise one's capacities, to explore, and to learn."* (Ryan & Deci 2000)

Intrinsic motivation is the internal desire to seek out new things and new challenges, whereas extrinsic motivation comes from influences outside of the individual (the carrot and stick approach, or rewards and punishments). Daniel Pink (2009) suggests that we are either extrinsically motivated (having an external reward or punishment for motivation) or intrinsically motivated (being self-motivated).

Students who are intrinsically motivated are more likely to engage in the task willingly and to work to improve their skills, which will increase their capabilities (Wigfield et al 2004). Pursuit of intrinsically motivated goals has been associated with improved wellbeing and mental health (Kasser & Ryan 1996) and reduced psychological distress (Ntoumanis & Standage 2009). When learning environments are supportive and nurturing, students tend to experience higher engagement (Norrish, Robinson & Williams 2011).

Self-determination theory (SDT)

Similarly, self-determination theory is concerned with the motivation behind the choices people make without external influence and interference (also known as extrinsic motivators.) SDT focuses on the degree to which an individual's behaviour is self-motivated and self-determined (Ryan & Deci 2017). We are most motivated in working towards intrinsic goals (Pink 2009).

The three needs for intrinsic motivation

SDT identifies three innate needs that, if satisfied, allow optimal function and growth:

1. Mastery – a belief that we can control outcomes through our actions and experience competence or mastery. We want to become a master at something.
2. Purpose – a sense of connection, relatedness, belonging, care, closeness and interaction with others. It's all about purpose and doing something meaningful beyond ourselves.
3. Autonomy – a level of independence, self-direction and being able to make choices and act in alignment with our own values (Ryan & Deci 2000; Pink 2009).

Fulfilment of these needs tends to lead us to being intrinsically motivated.

Enhancing intrinsic motivation

We can foster *mastery* by: exploring, understanding and cultivating strengths, and building on our existing skill sets.

We can foster *purpose* by: highlighting different areas of need and ways that students can help; fostering staff-student relationships; nurturing peer relationships and putting in place structures that encourage relationships like peer mentoring/buddy programs (Van Ryzin et al 2009).

We can foster *autonomy* by: allowing choice of activity; encouraging student voice and providing rationale for learning activities (Radel et al 2010).

A note about the intrinsic motivators of teachers

When students perceive a teacher to be intrinsically motivated to teach the class, the students themselves are more interested and involved (Radel et al 2010). This is a process of social contagion, whereby the influence of the teacher impacts the group. I propose that this is experienced as a result of mirror neurons, which are specialised brain cells that actually sense and then mimic (or mirror) the actions, feelings and sensations of another person (Iacoboni 2008). So one suggestion on building intrinsic motivation for students is to have motivated teachers (by building teacher mastery, purpose and autonomy).

This is obviously much harder to do in reality as most teachers will vary in their level of intrinsic motivation, particularly when it comes to teaching wellbeing, as many teachers perceive this lesson to be the 'last thing on their timetable' or the 'lowest value subject'. In this regard, most schools seem to follow the 20/60/20 rule whereby they have 20% of people who are keen and willing (early adopters), 60% who will go with the flow (early and late majority) and 20% who will struggle to come on board (laggards).

Each person's "willingness and ability to adopt an innovation depends on their awareness, interest and evaluation" (Rogers 2003). Keep in mind that their willingness and ability to adopt are not set in stone. If we can increase their awareness of why they should adopt, their interest in how it might help students and their evaluation of the effectiveness of implementation, they might be more willing.

Addressing inertia – sharing the small wins of early adopters
The other key consideration is the impact of inertia – in particular, that people can have a tendency to do nothing, or remain unchanged (some are more likely to do nothing than others)! If we can keep the changes simple (even easy) to do at first, that might be helpful for all members of our community. If we can find a small 'wedge' in order to get something started, it might be helpful. In particular, if we can have some small wins with our early adopters, who can share some of the success they have been having, that will be helpful (especially those early adopters who are held in high regard by the rest of the staff).

Also, if people are given the appropriate training, skills and resources to understand why they should adopt, as well as be able to adopt, this would be helpful. Doing this may actually increase teachers' intrinsic motivation, which will likely lead to higher engagement, involvement and participation from students in classrooms.

Discovering, developing and using character strengths

Strengths are ways of thinking, feeling and behaving that come naturally and easily to a person and which enable high functioning and performance (Linley & Harrington 2004). "Character strengths are the basic building blocks of goodness" (Niemiec et al 2013). While talents are valued for their tangible outcomes, character strengths are valued for moral or intrinsic reasons (Peterson & Seligman 2004).

Character strengths can be used to enhance wellbeing, overcome challenges and nurture relationships (Park, Peterson & Seligman 2004). In addition, by developing character strengths in our students, they become better equipped to make valuable contributions to society (Park & Peterson 2006).

Seligman and Peterson devised and validated the values in action (VIA) signature strengths survey, which measures 24 character strengths. This allows people to identify some of their key character strengths and use them accordingly.

The importance of using our strengths

When we have the opportunity to use our strengths (the things we are good at and enjoy doing), we are more likely to feel confident, creative, satisfied and engaged (McQuaid & Lawn 2014). Strengths are ways of thinking, feeling and behaving that come naturally and easily to us and enable high functioning and performance (Linley & Harrington 2004). When we work in our strengths – in our activities, relationships and learning – they energise us. We all have positive character traits to be discovered, valued, used and further developed.

Research has shown that using our top five strengths on a regular basis increases our wellbeing. These are referred to by Seligman and Peterson as our signature strengths. In particular, individuals who were able to use their signature strengths in new ways during a one-week trial were found to be happier and less depressed at one month and six month follow-ups (Seligman, Steen & Peterson 2005). Furthermore, individuals who use their strengths tend to report greater vitality and psychological wellbeing, they make more progress towards their goals (Linley et al 2010) and experience enhanced resilience after stressful events (Peterson & Seligman 2003).

Character strengths and our negativity bias

One reason that character strengths are so powerful for wellbeing is due to our negativity bias. As mentioned in Section 2 on positive emotion, we have a tendency to focus on negative stimuli more strongly than positive stimuli, thereby making us more aware of our weaknesses and flaws than our strengths (Baumeister et al 2001). Furthermore, because we so consistently act with our strengths, we are often not consciously aware of them and this creates a blind spot (Biswas-Diener et al 2010). So, it is not surprising that identifying, articulating and intentionally developing our strengths contributes positively to our wellbeing.

A list of character strengths

The 24 character strengths can be characterised under six broad areas, known as virtues. These are:

Virtues	Character Strengths
Wisdom and Knowledge	Creativity, Curiosity, Open-mindedness, Love of Learning and Perspective
Courage	Honesty, Bravery, Persistence and Zest
Humanity	Kindness, Love and Social Intelligence
Justice	Fairness, Leadership and Teamwork
Temperance	Forgiveness, Modesty, Prudence and Self-regulation)
Transcendence	Appreciation of Beauty And Excellence, Gratitude, Hope, Humour and Religiousness/Spirituality

(Peterson & Seligman 2004).

Character strength surveys

You can take the online survey and find out more about these specific character strengths at http://www.viacharacter.org/www/#nav.

A youth survey, as well as an adult survey, have been developed in order to help people aged 13 and over engage in a process of self-examination of their own strengths. Once the survey has been completed, respondents are provided with their character strengths profile, listing (ranking) their strengths from 1 to 24 according to their responses. This represents a suitable starting point for applying and evolving these strengths further.

A character-strengths approach can be implemented with staff and students; it will lead to increased self-awareness and awareness of others. Teachers should first identify their own strengths and how they could utilise them more on a daily basis. Teachers can then implement a similar process with students. Useful suggestions for how each strength could be applied is available on the VIA (Values in Action) Strengths website (2019).

Overusing our character strengths

It is possible to consider each strength on a continuum, in which too much of a strength in a particular context becomes overuse, too little is underuse, and the centre area is the 'strengths zone' or optimal expression of the strength. From this perspective, "when a strength is overused, it is no longer a strength" (Niemic 2014). For example, too much modesty might be self-deprecation; too much curiosity might come across as being a 'nosy parker', too much bravery could lead to unhealthy risk-taking.

Strengths are flexible

Our character is made up of lots of different strengths that we have developed in our lives, and as a result, everyone has a different set of strengths. There seems to me to be a lot of work being done by schools in this area (many seem to make it their first focus in Positive Education), although I think that sometimes this may result in slightly unhelpful and unintended messages that come about with a 'strengths-based approach'.

In particular, it is important that we don't consider our strengths to be inherent and unchanging parts of our character. We should instead avoid rigid conceptions of ourselves and consider our strengths as capable of being improved (Dweck 2006). James Anderson (2018) says, "there's nothing wrong with building on your strengths, as long as it's not at the expense of believing you couldn't be building on your weaknesses." We are in fact able to build on our strengths *and* our weaknesses. Strengths are indeed flexible and able to be adapted.

Strengths Summary

The research does however, support a strengths-based approach in schools, informing us that when we choose to build on our strengths (rather than our weaknesses) we will tend to increase positive development and thriving (Peterson & Park 2009). Knowing our strengths and using them every day can lead to increased performance, as well as feeling more confident and satisfied with life. They are the things we are good at and enjoy doing (McQuaid & Lawn 2014). Using and developing our strengths allows us to help our brain perform at its best (Buckingham & Clifton 2001).

We can also encourage our students to begin to articulate their own strengths and those of others. Our team thoroughly enjoy leading students through a process of giving "shout-outs" during our incursions- whereby students are given the opportunity to affirm someone else in the group for their awesome conduct and contribution. Very powerful. You can also find a modified version in this in Part 2 of this book in the PWP's.

It is clear from the research that identifying and applying our character strengths every day contributes to our wellbeing. In practice, schools are already equipped to lead a focused process of learning about character strengths in order to help the whole community on its journey of thriving.

Practices to build Engagement

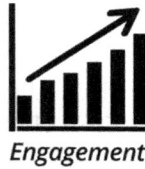

Engagement

ENGAGEMENT	
Find a way to play	Each day, take a little time to be silly, not serious. Have a joke, dance with your kids, do a cartwheel. Just be light and create a space to let go, if only for a moment.
Strengths reflection	At the end of each day, make a note in your journal about how you were able to use one of your signature strengths during the day.
Stand up regularly	If you are working at a desk, be sure to stand up and move every 20-30 minutes. It is likely to improve creativity, productivity and wellbeing.
Take a strengths pause	Between the activities of your day, take a couple of breaths and then ask yourself, "Which of my strengths will I bring forward now?"
Your superhero strengths	Think of a time when you have been proud of yourself. Reflect on what personal character strengths you used to get to that point. Write about this in your journal. *PWP Wk 36

Savouring the moment	Find something to savour right now in the present moment. Use your senses to find something that you are experiencing now that is enjoyable. It might be the sound of a bird outside, the sunshine or breeze coming in through a window or just relaxing and sitting quietly. Simply notice it, be present and appreciate it. *PWP Wk 31
Intrinsic motivation	Identify one instance in your life where you have used intrinsic motivation, fuelled by purpose, autonomy and mastery. Write about this in your journal. *PWP Wk 16
Me at my best	Think of a time when you have been at your best (when you have been the best possible version of yourself). Now write briefly about this time when you were at your best, and identify the strengths you used. *PWP Wk 10
Flow activity	Consider when you were last so engaged in an activity, that you lost track of time. Consider investing some time this weekend engaging in that activity. *PWP Wk 8
* For more information and to lead this practice with your students, go to the relevant PWP in Part 2.	

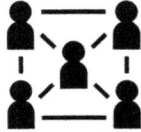

Relationships

> *"Friendships multiply joy and divide grief."* – Swedish Proverb
>
> *"The only thing that really matters in life are your relationships to other people."* – George Vaillant

Our relationships with other people matter. Secure relationships tend to consist of kindness to self and others; a sense of belonging; humility, forgiveness, gratitude; authenticity and honesty. After analysing many studies on happiness over the last few decades, researchers have concluded that "like food and air, we seem to need social relationships to thrive" (Diener & Biswas-Diener 2008).

Relationships and oxytocin

Researchers have found the factor that distinguished the happiest 10 percent of people from everyone else was the strength of their social relationships (Diener & Seligman 2002). When we make positive social connections, our body releases oxytocin – a pleasure inducing chemical – into our bloodstream. Oxytocin is sometimes referred to as 'the love drug', as it plays a role in bonding, friendships and orgasms. This is why we can seem to be 'in sync' or connected to certain people. Furthermore, oxytocin also reduces our anxiety, improves our concentration and focus and helps to regulate our cardiovascular system.

Relationships provide support

Social support and positive school relationships provide a buffer in difficult times. These strong social supports are linked to better academic performance (Wentzell & Caldwell 1997), along with adolescent wellbeing and resilience (Cohen & Wills 1985; Stewart et al 2004).

Seligman (2002) states that "relationships are the best antidote to the downs of life, and the single most reliable up." If children and adolescents feel included and accepted, particularly by a larger peer group, they are more likely to feel positive about themselves (Berndt 1992; Hartup 2002). Limited social connectedness is a risk factor for depression, substance abuse, suicide and work related stress (Hassed 2008; Achor 2010). It seems that investing in a healthy social support network is one of the best things we can do to enhance our own thriving. In schools, cultivating respectful relationships for all members of our community is essential.

Unhealthy relationships

It is important to consider the possible negative effects of relationships. In particular, some relationships are critical or abusive (Hawker & Boulton 2000), while others are associated with peer pressure and risk taking behaviours (Maxwell 2002). Sometimes, our need for relationships can mean that we choose to hang on to unhealthy relationships, instead of experiencing isolation (Myers 2000).

Students who only have a few key relationships at school may be more prone to hanging onto them, even if they are unhealthy. This highlights the need to help students to understand healthy relationships and develop the skills for nurturing them.

Building relationships

A few useful concepts we can use to build our relationships are active-constructive responding, forgiveness, self-compassion, emotional bank accounts and the platinum rule.

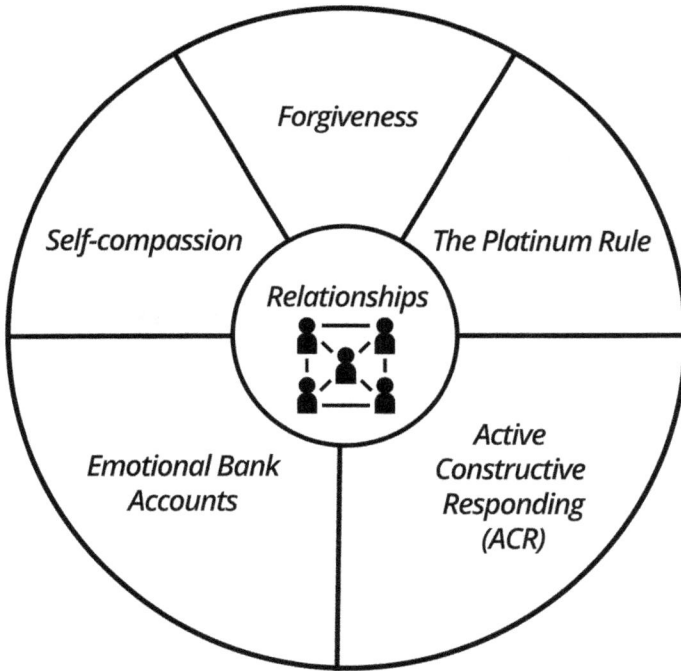

Active Constructive Responding (ACR)

Some young (and not so young) people lack critical social skills that enable them to build healthy relationships. Active constructive responding refers to the way that we respond when someone is sharing something positive with us. How we respond to the good news of others can either build a relationship or undermine it (Gable, Gonzaga & Strachman 2006). It can be a useful model for sharing with young people and provides them with a useful tool for enhancing their relationships.

4 ways to respond	
Active constructive responding (to encourage/ build).	**Passive constructive responding (to minimise).**
Active destructive responding (to point out the negative).	**Passive destructive responding (to brush off or ignore).**

ACR involves responding by offering interest, enthusiasm, support, encouragement and sometimes follow-up questions when someone shares good news. I have also found it to be a useful tool for my own relationships and one that I continue to work on to build better relationships and connections. It is my opinion that in many cases 2 minutes of active constructive responding is as beneficial to a relationship as six months without it.

Personal benefits of ACR
- Increased positive emotions
- Increased subjective wellbeing
- Increased self-esteem
- Decreased loneliness

Relationship benefits of ACR
- Increased relationship/marital satisfaction
- Increased intimacy
- Increased commitment
- Increased trust, liking, closeness
- Increased stability

(Gable & Reis 2010)

Using ACR – an example

Below is a hypothetical scenario that demonstrates four different ways of responding to someone who is sharing good news. ACR benefits the individual we are relating to as well as the relationship itself. Conversely, each of the other three types has been shown to have a negative impact on the wellbeing of those sharing the good news and also on the relationship (Gable, Gonzaga & Strachman 2006).

Situation: A husband responds to his wife's news that she is being considered for a promotion.

Active constructive responding (to encourage/build).	"That is wonderful! I am so happy for you. You would be excellent in that new position." (Responding enthusiastically; maintaining eye contact, smiling, displaying positive emotions.)
Active destructive responding (to point out the negative).	"If you get the promotion, you are going to have to be at work all week and on Saturday mornings, too." (Pointing out the downside; displaying negative nonverbal cues.)
Passive constructive responding (to minimise).	"That's nice that you are being considered for the promotion." (Happy, but lacking enthusiasm/ downplaying; little to no active emotional expression.)
Passive destructive responding (to brush off or ignore).	"A promotion, huh? Well, hurry up and get changed so we can get some dinner. I'm starving." (Lacking interest, displaying little to no eye contact, turning away, leaving the room.)

(Magyar-Moe 2009)

Strengthening ACR

ACR is a skill, and just like any other it can be developed with practice. During some of our incursions we offer for students, students are guided through this process. Using our PWP's, you may also do that in a way that builds students understanding of ACR and which gives them time to reflect and record their own responses and then to make adjustments over a period of time. It will enhance their relationships and wellbeing and ultimately will help them thrive.

Forgiveness

The Greek translation of the work "forgiveness" literally means "to let go." Forgiveness is "conceptualized as the process of making peace with life. When we are able to forgive another person, oneself, or a situation/circumstance, we are capable of freeing ourselves from a negative association to the source" (Raj et al 2016).

Forgiveness is not pardoning, condoning or excusing the behaviour and does not always mean reconciliation (Lyubomirsky 2008). When we forgive, we don't need to forget, but we do need to choose not to let previous actions (of ourselves or others) control our present or future actions or emotions. Forgiveness is an important part of good relationships, and it enhances physical and psychological wellbeing.

Benefits of forgiveness

Studies show that more forgiving people differ significantly to less forgiving people on many personality attributes. Forgiving people are found to be less ruminative, (Metts & Cupach 1998) less narcissistic (Davidson 1993), less exploitative and more empathic (Tangney et al 1999) than less forgiving people.

Forgiveness and mental health

Forgiveness was also found to be positively connected to global mental health and relationship quality (Berry & Worthington 2001) and hope

(Rye et al 2000) and was correlated with lower anxiety and depression among college students (Al-Mabuk & Enright 1995). High self-esteem and low levels of anxiety and depression were the results of higher levels of forgiveness among elderly women (Hebl & Enright 1993). Parents who were high on forgiveness were also high on self-esteem and positive parenting styles (Al-Mabuk & Enright 1995).

Indicators of forgiveness

There are many benefits of being able to forgive. One factor that indicates someone's willingness to forgive is positive emotions. In particular, "positive emotions contribute to the ability for the individuals to recover from negative emotional experiences of transgression" (Raj et al 2016).

A second indicator of forgiveness is the modelling that young people find in "parents and other influential people, such as teachers in school and religious institutions" (Raj et al 2016). So parents, teachers and schools would do well to both model forgiveness in their own lives, but also to espouse the virtue of forgiveness. At UPP, we help schools lead students through this process through some of our incursions, or through our PWP's.

Self-compassion

Compassion is "sympathetic concern for the sufferings or mis-fortunes of others" (Oxford Dictionary 2018). So often, we are compassionate towards others, and yet we don't offer ourselves the same level of concern. "Self-compassion involves treating yourself with the same kindness, concern and support you would show to a good friend. When faced with difficult life struggles, or confronting personal mistakes, failures and inadequacies, self-compassion responds with kindness rather than harsh self-judgment, recognizing that imperfection is part of the shared human experience" (Neff & Dahm 2015).

The importance of self-compassion

Research suggests that higher levels of self-kindness are associated with greater optimism, compassion, forgiveness and goal mastery, as well as lower rates of anxiety, self-criticism and perfectionism (Niemiec 2017; Neff & McGehee 2010; Neff & Pommier 2013). When we are kind to ourselves, it feels good, and that positive emotion helps us to be more outward facing, better at problem solving and critical thinking and more creative (Fredrickson 2001). When we experience self-kindness, we're more likely to feel social connection (Niemiec 2017). Self-kindness is strongly associated with wellbeing amongst adolescents and adults (Neff & McGehee 2010).

To look at it another way, if you treated a friend the way you sometimes treat yourself, would you still be friends?

Six tips for self-compassion

Carla Ford (2018) offers us her six tips for self-kindness:

1. Carve out time for yourself to do something that feels good – go for a coffee, have a bath, read a good book; do something that brings you joy.
2. Notice your self-talk, and cut yourself some slack. Everybody makes mistakes and nobody is perfect. Speak to yourself as you would a friend.
3. Discover JOMO (the joy of missing out) and give social media a miss for a while. Everybody posts their best selves and it can make us feel bad that our lives don't match up. Be kind and have a day free of social comparison.
4. Acknowledge your successes. We're always quick to do that for others, so why not take a few minutes and consider all you've achieved?
5. Hang out with your cheerleaders. Spend time with the people who uplift you and support you – the ones who fill your tank.

6. Take your daily 'MEDS' (Mindfulness, Exercise, Diet and Sleep). Looking after your mind and body is a great form of self-kindness.

Emotional Bank Accounts

Stephen Covey uses the metaphor of *Emotional Bank Accounts* (EBA) to describe "the amount of trust that's been built up in a relationship" (1989). The basic tenet of this simple yet profound principle is that we maintain a personal emotional bank account with anyone who relates with us. The EBA begins on a neutral balance. And just as with any bank account, we can make deposits and withdrawals. However, instead of dealing with units of monetary value, we deal with emotional units.

Relationships are our accumulation of interactions – the sum of these parts reflects the health of the relationship (Fredrickson 2013). Our relationships are the sum of our deposits, less our withdrawals. Although, I propose that our withdrawals might be more noticeable by others than our deposits (as a result of our negativity bias).

There are two other ways to explain this – Gottman's 'magic ratio' (2002) and Rath and Clifton's (2004) 'bucket and dipper' theory. Each will be explained briefly in this section.

The 'magic ratio' of social interactions
Thanks to John Gottman's pioneering research on marriages, we now understand that the frequency of small, positive acts is critical. He suggests there is a 'magic ratio' in terms of our balance of positive to negative interactions. After studying over 700 married couples during 15-minute interactions, he had a 94% success rate in predicting divorce.

In particular, Gottman found that marriages are significantly more likely to succeed when the couple's interactions are near a 5 to 1 ratio of positive to negative. When the ratio approaches 1 to 1, marriages tend to "cascade to divorce" (Gottman 2002). It is suggested that in all of our other relationships in our lives (at work or in our personal lives), the Losada ratio of 2.9 to 1 (or better), will reflect a healthy relationship (Losada & Heaphy 2004).

The 'bucket and dipper' theory of social interactions

Another way to look at this concept is that of Tom Rath and Don Clifton (2004) who share the 'bucket and dipper' theory. They say that "each one of us has an invisible bucket. It is constantly emptied or filled, depending on what others say or do to us. When our bucket is full, we feel great. When it is empty, we feel awful.

Each of us also has an invisible dipper. When we use that dipper to fill other people's buckets by saying or doing things to increase their positive emotions, we also fill our own bucket. But when we use that dipper to dip from others' buckets by doing or saying things that decrease their positive emotions, we diminish ourselves."

In the same way that we can fill others' buckets and be mindful of our positive interactions to attain that magic ratio in our relationships, we can consider ways to make deposits into the EBAs that we share with others.

Making deposits or withdrawals

Some ways to build into the emotional bank balance of others (and make deposits) are:

- Mindfully pay attention instead of ignoring.
- Hold a stress reducing conversation (undivided attention when the goal is to express understanding of the other person's feelings and perspective).

- Communicate understanding, rather than trying to solve the problem. (Note – the author's wife wishes he would take his own medicine and do more of this one. Luckily, she understands that he is a work in progress and that progress is sometimes slow!)
- Apologise when we make withdrawals.
- Make deposits each day.
- Listen (seeking first to understand, then to be understood).
- Be kind, polite and considerate of the needs of others.
- Take turns, share and include others.
- Smile and offer a greeting.
- Help and serve others.
- Bring positive energy.
- Be polite and considerate.
- Compliment others or express gratitude for something they have done.
- Recognise and show appreciation to others for their behaviour/ achievements.
- Be generous.
- Speak words of affirmation daily: compliments or words of encouragement (at UPP, we call these shout-outs).
- Invest quality time: give your partner undivided attention.
- Give gifts: symbols of love, like flowers or chocolates.
- Perform acts of service: set the table, walk the dog or do other small jobs.
- Engage in physical touch: holding hands, kissing, hugging.

(Rath & Clifton 2004; Chapman 1992; Covey 1989; Algoe, Haidt & Gable 2008; Gottman 2002).

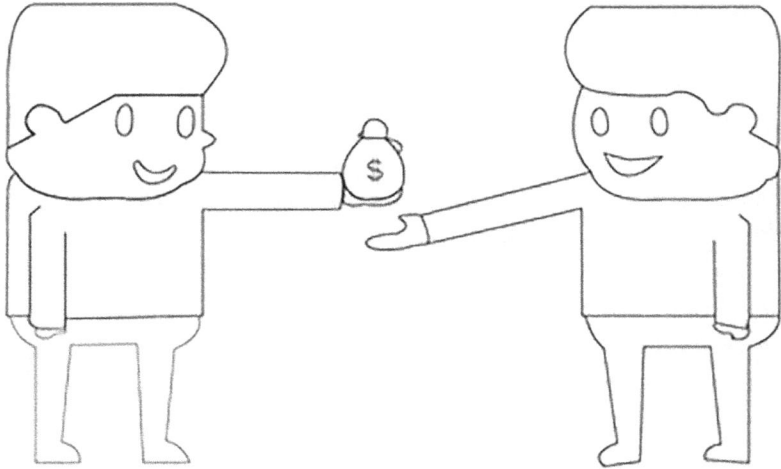

We make withdrawals from our EBAs when we:
- Make fun of someone
- Do or say mean things
- Ignore someone
- Bully or criticise
- Physically hurt someone
- Are sarcastic, cynical or show disapproval (Losada & Heaphy 2004).

Reciprocity of social interactions

The good news is when we make a deposit, we will often be repaid in kind. This social norm of responding to a positive action with another positive action, rewarding kind actions, is called reciprocity. Reciprocity means that in response to friendly actions, people are frequently much nicer and much more cooperative than predicted by the self-interest model. Conversely, in response to hostile actions people are frequently much more nasty and even brutal than expected (Fehr & Gachter 2000).

According to this research, if you are quite kind to someone, they will on average pay you back with a little more kindness than you showed to them. As St Francis of Assisi once said, "It is in giving that we receive." Or another way to look at it is, "What goes around comes around." So if you can't be kind for the benefit of others, it might be wise to be kind to others for your own benefit.

It is impossible to make a withdrawal and a deposit simultaneously. But it is wise to consider that what one person considers a deposit, is not necessarily a deposit for everyone. This can be explained by the platinum rule.

The Platinum Rule

How might they like to be treated?

If you were making biscuits for someone in your kitchen, it would be wise to consider the sort of biscuits *they* would like to eat (choc chip, Anzacs, shortbread etc). Don't make your favourite ones to give to them if they don't like them.

In the same way, if we are being intentional about investing in our EBA with someone in our lives, individualisation is the key, as people differ in the way they like to be treated. How do they like their biscuits? Instead of the golden rule – "treat others as *you* would like to be treated" – the platinum rule suggests that we might instead "treat others as *they* would like to be treated."

Have you ever received a gift from someone (for a birthday or anniversary, etc) that you didn't particularly want? In these cases, we can usually appreciate the gesture, but not the actual gift. In these cases, we may even take the gift back to the shop and replace it with something else.

Similarly, sometimes we may attempt to make deposits, but our efforts don't quite hit the spot. It is important that our efforts are aligned with the preferences of the receiver. How do they want to be treated? So consider the other person and what they would actually consider a deposit in their emotional bank account. It's no good paying them in Australian dollars if they like to spend Japanese yen!

Practices to build relationships

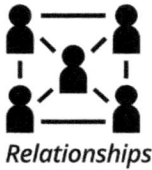

Relationships

RELATIONSHIPS	
Offer micro moves	Practise compassion by offering to help someone with their workload (when you notice they are struggling) or check in to see if they are managing everything that's on their plate.
Do a 5-minute favour	Spend five minutes each week helping someone in your network (at home or work). Share information, make a recommendation or help a neighbour/colleague carry something from the car instead of them making two trips.
Forgiveness	Do a loving-kindness meditation. First, focus on yourself. Secondly, focus on someone who you are holding some grudge or resentment towards. The mantra is as follows:

	May (I) they be well, May (I) they be happy, May (I) they be peaceful, May (I) they let go of anger and sadness. *PWP Wk 39
Kindness catching	Think of (and write down) three times that you have been kind to others in the past. Record as much detail as you can. *PWP Wk 38
Active constructive responding	The next time you are in a social setting, practise responding in an active, constructive way. Listen, give eye contact and show interest in the person speaking by asking questions and being encouraging. *PWP Wk 13
Shout-outs!	When you arrive at work each morning, send an email to compliment a colleague on the quality of their work that you witnessed. Or share this compliment in person when you notice someone in your life demonstrate a quality that you value. *PWP Wk 12 & PWP Wk 40
Act of kindness	Spend a few moments thinking of something good you can do for someone today. Then act on it. *PWP Wk 11
* For more information and to lead this practice with your students, go to the relevant PWP in Part 2.	

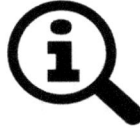

Meaning

> *"He who has a why to live for can bear almost any how."*
> – Friedrich Nietzsche
>
> *"Having a clear sense of meaning and purpose contributes to 'the will to live' when placed in extreme life-threatening situations."*
> – Viktor Frankl
>
> *"A person without purpose is like a ship without a rudder."*
> – Thomas Carlisle.
>
> *"The best way to find yourself is to lose yourself in the service of others."*
> – Mahatma Gandhi

Meaning in the Wellbeing and Positive Education context refers to "understanding, believing in and serving something greater than yourself, and deliberately engaging in activities for the benefits of others" (Norrish, Robinson & Williams 2011). Meaning is defined as "having a sense of where one fits in the world" (Steger et al 2008). It consists of three parts:

a) Understanding and accepting ourselves
b) Understanding the world around us
c) Understanding where we fit within the world and with others

A meaningful life

While fame and glamour are about the self, leading a meaningful life is about connecting and contributing to something bigger (Smith 2017). Victor Frankl (1992) proposes in his book 'Man's Search for Meaning' that humans have an innate drive to experience their life as meaningful. It matters to us, whether we matter or not. This need for meaning leads to a strong and resilient life.

It is a noble aim for schools to instil a sense of responsibility for the world we live in and a commitment to helping others. This sense of meaning or purpose will not only help the world and others, it will also help those who engage in its pursuit.

In particular, purposelessness is a risk factor for depression, risk taking behaviours, poor social relationships, substance abuse, suicidal ideation and alcohol use (Kim et al 2017; Damon et al 2003). However, those with a stronger sense of purpose tend to engage in more protective health behaviours, experience more positive emotions, enjoy greater happiness and life satisfaction, higher levels of physical and mental health and greater sense of control in their lives (Battersby & Phillips 2016; Hassed 2008). In adolescents, purpose can be viewed as a defining feature of wellbeing.

Being clear on our purpose in life is also linked to having more resilience, an ability to bounce back despite difficulty and the ability to pursue goals despite hardships (McKnight & Kashdan 2009).

On a related note, Angela Duckworth's (2007) definition of grit is "perseverance and passion for long-term goals". Note the use of the word passion – if we are passionate about something, we are far more likely to make sacrifices and work towards it. Similarly, if we can see the underlying meaning or purpose behind something, we will be more likely to stick with it when problems arise.

The need to 'start with why'

Simon Sinek (2011) highlights the need to 'start with why' – in particular referring to the need for us to identify why we are doing something. If our why (our purpose or meaning) is strong, we are more likely to prevail.

The meaningful life consists of belonging to and serving something that we believe is bigger than ourselves (Seligman 2011). We usually draw meaning from multiple sources, including family and love, work, religion and various personal projects (Emmons 1997). To find meaning we need to look for the positive difference we are making for others in our daily lives.

Fostering purpose in our students

The search for meaning during adolescence is considered to be adaptive and beneficial. However, a search for meaning that commences later in life can often be quite distressing and is often related to lower wellbeing and satisfaction with life (Bronk et al 2009).

If this is the case, how can we help foster a sense of meaning or purpose in our students? Encouraging young people to participate in activities such as helping at home, volunteering in the community, faith-related activities or engaging in the arts can precipitate the development of meaning. However, these activities should not be ad-hoc and there should also be the opportunity to reflect on the meaning derived from them (Fry 1998; Bronk 2014).

Finally, engaging young people in focused discussion about what matters to them – their personal values and aspirations – can assist them in the development of longer-term, authentic goals. The correlation between meaning and optimal wellbeing provides a convincing case for it to be explored in schools. After all, what more can we want our young people to aspire to than a life which has direction, which is meaningful to them and in which they leverage their strengths to make a positive contribution to the world?

Ways to explore meaning

Some ways to explore meaning are through ikigai; kindness and altruism; and spirituality.

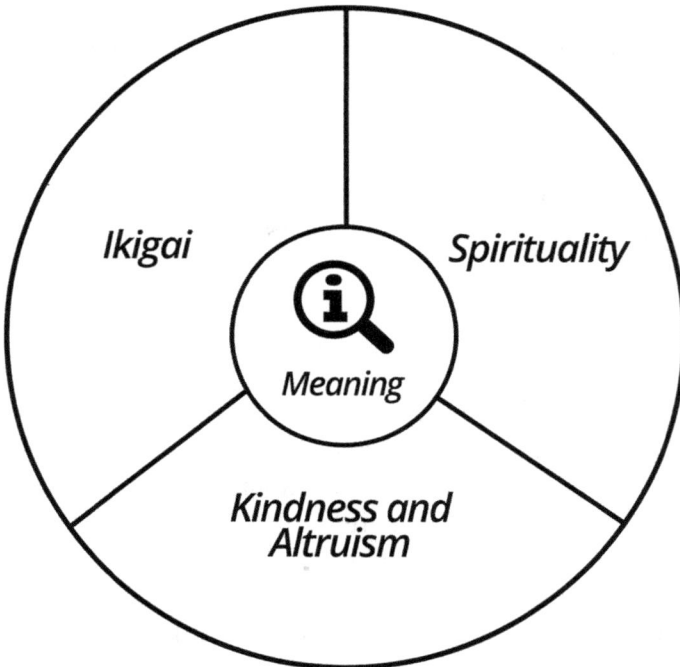

Ikigai

Ikigai is a Japanese word which translates roughly to *a reason for being*, encompassing joy, a sense of purpose and meaning and a feeling of wellbeing. Its two parts – *iki,* meaning life and *kai,* meaning *the realisation of hopes and expectations* (Better Humans 2017) but it also has the nuance of "the reason for which you wake up in the morning" (The Ascent 2018). Each individual's ikigai is personal to them and specific to their lives, values and beliefs. Activities that allow one to feel ikigai are never forced on an individual; they are often spontaneous and always undertaken willingly, giving the individual satisfaction and a sense of meaning to life (Nakanishi 1999).

Ikigai involves asking four key questions and identifying what responses may lie close to the centre of the diagram for a particular person.
- What do you love?
- What are you good at?
- What can you be paid for?
- What does the world need?

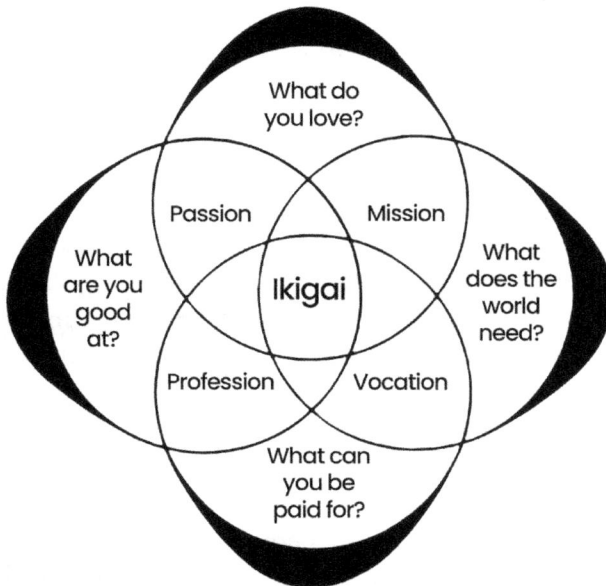

Howard Thurman famously said "don't ask yourself what the world needs. Ask yourself what makes you come alive and then go do that. Because what the world needs is people who have come alive." In light of ikigai, it might be appropriate to ask both of those questions and find where our answers intersect.

Kindness and Altruism

"Altruism is a benevolent state of mind concerned more with loving than being loved." – Aristotle 350 BC

"Never give up on giving." – Stephen Post

"Meaning is directly concerned with doing things for others." – John Hendry

"Everything that lives, lives not alone, nor for itself." – William Blake

"Life is not meaningful unless it is serving an end beyond itself, unless it is of value to someone else." – Abraham Joshua Heschel

Professor Jane Dutton explains that we all have a psychological need to feel respected, valued and appreciated. As we saw in the previous section, relationships with other people are important. Investing into a healthy support network is one of the best things we can do to enhance our own wellbeing. Helping and being kind to others improves our connectedness and makes us happier (Lyubomirsky 2007).

The value of being kind

Kindness is good for us and it can come in many forms. One research study focused on generosity of time (volunteering), money (charity) and in relationships (emotional availability and hospitality). The study surveyed 2,000 people over five years.

It found that those people who were more generous were happier, less depressed and healthier. In particular, those who described themselves as 'very happy' volunteered an average of almost six hours per month, while those who are 'unhappy' volunteered an average of less than 40 mins per month (Smith & Davidson 2014).

In addition, depression rates were lower for those participants who donated more than 10 percent of their incomes to charity. And finally, those who were more generous in their relationships (emotionally available and hospitable to others) were much more likely to be in excellent health (48 percent) than those who were not (31 percent). I would argue that many of the people who give time and money are in a position to do so (which would likely make them happier than those who are not in a position to do so). However, there would also be many people who are in a position to give, who do not do so willingly.

A very powerful way for us to foster more kindness in our lives is to think of times that we ourselves have been kind to others. In a study done by Adam Grant at Wharton Business school (2013), people who were asked to remember the times that they themselves had been kind gave more generously to others than those people who were asked to remember times when others had been kind to them. Recalling our actions of kindness helps us reinforce and build a vivid self-image of ourselves as a kind person. We then find ways to live up to the 'kind person' image and become more kind.

Kindness and generosity are contagious

In addition to increasing happiness and health and reducing depression, generosity has been found to be contagious. Receiving help increases the likelihood of being generous towards a stranger. Researchers have found that when we receive an act of kindness, we are quite likely to 'pay it forward' (Tsvetkova & Macy 2014; Jordan et al 2013).

In essence, when we demonstrate kindness towards someone, it is quite possible that the flow-on effect of our generosity will be much larger than the small generous act we offer. It may, in fact, be passed on. One such report occurred in December 2012, when someone bought a coffee at a drive-thru window (Tim Horton's Coffee Shop) and paid for their own coffee as well as for the person in the car behind them. The next customer paid for the car behind them, and so on, and for the next three hours a total of 228 customers did this (Mallough 2013).

Other such instances of between four and 24 cars paying it forward have been reported by Wendy's, McDonald's, Starbucks, Del Taco, Taco Bell, KFC and Dunkin' Donuts restaurants across the USA (Tsvetkova & Macy 2014). If it's possible in the USA, it's probable in our lucky country! Generosity has been called contagious, probably as a result of situations like this. When we experience generosity, there seems to be a willingness to pass it on.

Toddlers spontaneously develop kindness behaviours and appear to experience happiness when being kind to others (Warneken et al 2006; Ankin et al 2012). Kindness has also been shown to help buffer against the negative effects of stress and trauma (Niemiec 2017). It has already been well established that compassion, love and social support have health benefits for recipients (Ainsworth et al 1978; Harlow 1958).

A positive feedback loop

A positive feedback loop exists between spending money on others (i.e. prosocial spending) and happiness. Participants recalled a previous purchase made for either themselves or someone else and then reported their happiness. Afterward, participants chose whether to spend a monetary windfall on themselves or someone else.

Participants assigned to recall a purchase made for someone else reported feeling significantly happier immediately after this recollection. Most importantly, the happier participants felt, the more likely they were to choose to spend a windfall on someone else in the near future. Thus, by providing initial evidence for a positive feedback loop between prosocial spending and wellbeing, this data offers one potential path to sustainable happiness: prosocial spending increases happiness, which in turn encourages prosocial spending (Ankin, Dunn & Norton 2012).

Volunteering might contribute to happiness levels by increasing empathic emotions and shifting aspirations (Borgonovi 2008). Results indicate that altruistic attitudes, volunteering and informal helping behaviours are related to life satisfaction and positive affect (Kahana et al 2013) as well as wellbeing, happiness, health and longevity. This holds true so long as we are not overwhelmed by helping tasks (Post 2005). That is, if we are feeling depleted and we are inundated with an expectation to help, that may not be beneficial.

The bystander effect

Interestingly, while *experiencing* generosity increases our likelihood of being generous, *observing* generous acts directed towards others can lead us to believe that our generosity is no longer needed. As a result, we can be less generous because of what researchers call 'the bystander effect' – the typical 'someone else will do it' syndrome (Tsvetkova & Macy 2014). Therefore, if we are to spread our generosity, it may be worth investigating ways of being generous in private, rather than in public and so avoiding 'the bystander effect'.

Applications

In schools, this can be created into a small project for students – they might be invited to find one totally unselfish thing to do for someone else who needs a hand. Not only does this benefit the receiver and the giver of generosity – it can spark a generosity cycle within a school (or within a small pocket of the school – e.g. a year level, house group or classroom).

Targeted acts of kindness

Random acts of kindness are often suggested; however, I am of the opinion that it need not be 'random' to have the desired impact. For me, random acts of kindness seem a little superficial and are often more centred around the person doing the giving. Instead, I believe that 'targeted' acts of kindness move us from a focus on ourselves to meeting a genuine need for someone who may require it. These acts are much more personal and meaningful. They are more responsive – we keep an open mind to spot a need; then we do what we can to meet that need.

Targeted acts of kindness can still be done in private. However, they require us to be more intentional about choosing a person and tailoring our generosity towards something that is of value to them. Or we could choose to be aware of the world around us – on the lookout to identify a need that we can help with. We might encourage our students to "never see a need without doing something about it" as St Mary MacKillop urged people to do.

In any case (random or targeted), generosity has benefits for our school community and can contribute to the wellbeing of both staff and students. As parents and educators, it is also helpful on a personal level. Not only should we teach this to kids, we should live it ourselves.

Spirituality

Spirituality is "the quality of being concerned with the human spirit or soul as opposed to material or physical things" (Oxford

Dictionary 2018). Spirituality represents internal beliefs and values, whereas religiousness represents the outwards expression of such beliefs, including religious practices, rituals and traditions (Cotton et al 2005).

Spirituality has a protective influence against at risk behaviours (substance abuse, sexual promiscuity); a positive impact on coping with bereavement and illness; and mental health benefits, such as reduced depressive symptoms (Cotton, et al 2005). Spirituality (independent of religious denomination) also seems to be linked to physical and mental wellbeing. Researchers propose that one of the main reasons for this is that religious communities tend to be a source of social support and connectedness, as well as positive shared community behaviours (Hassed 2008).

It would also seem that spirituality contributes to a greater sense of meaning and purpose in life (Steger & Frazier 2005). The sharp increase in youth suicide may well be related to the turning away from the search for spirituality among young people (Dervic et al 2004).

While the influence of spirituality on health is not always easy to determine, the evidence points to it having an important role in the prevention and management of a range of psychological and physical illnesses (Koenig 2001; Townsend et al 2002), as well as helping one to cope, especially with chronic and life-threatening conditions (Sullivan 2003).

Practices to build meaning

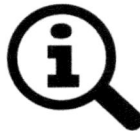

Meaning

MEANING	
Volunteer playground duty	Volunteer to take your colleague's playground duty.
For the sake of what?	Spend five minutes writing what you would be willing to get out of your comfort zone for or to risk failure for.
Get spiritual	Take time to connect with a cause greater than yourself. Pause, connect, pray, think and reflect, in whatever way is helpful to you.
Be awed by nature	Get outside whenever you can. Try to soak it up by noticing and being mindful of your surroundings, with all five senses.
Awe-inspiring	Think of a time that you have experienced an awe-inspiring moment – a time when you witnessed beauty in the world. It could be in nature, in a museum, an act of moral courage or kindness, music, art or a person's story that inspired you. Share this moment with someone else. *PWP Wk 25

Live your legacy	Write a brief summary of how you would personally like to be remembered and described, using some values, personal characteristics and contributions to humanity that really stand out for you. Start living your legacy now. *PWP Wk 24
Make the mundane meaningful	The next time you are doing a task that you find relatively meaningless, consider "How could this task possibly help me in the future, or how could it help someone or something else?" *PWP Wk 23
* For more information and to lead this practice with your students, go to the relevant PWP in Part 2.	

Section 6 – Accomplishment

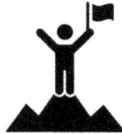

Accomplishment

Accomplishment can be defined as "a thing done successfully with effort, skill or courage" (Oxford 2018). It is the "development of individual potential through setting for and achieving meaningful outcomes" (Norrish, Robinson & Williams 2011).

'Need for achievement' refers to an individual's desire for significant accomplishment, mastering of skills, or high standards (Murray 1938). The need for achievement can be associated with a range of actions, including "intense, prolonged and repeated efforts to accomplish something difficult. To work with singleness of purpose towards a high and distant goal. To have the determination to win."

The accomplishment of worthwhile goals has been found to lead to positive emotions and wellbeing (Sheldon et al 2010).

In order to explore this topic, we will focus on goal theory, hope theory, growth mindset and grit.

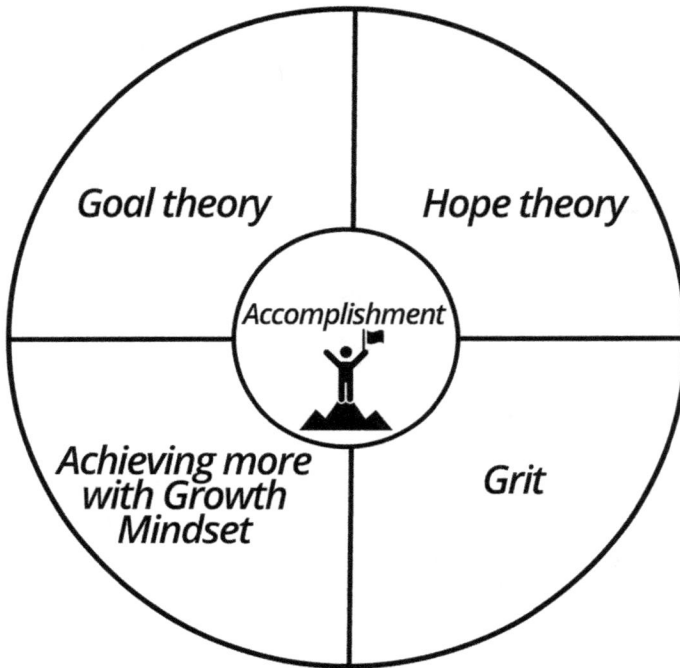

Goal theory

A goal is an idea of the future or desired result that a person or a group of people envisions, plans and commits to achieve (Locke & Latham 1990).

According to Locke and Latham, the fathers of goal setting theory (2002), goals affect performance in the following ways:
1. goals direct attention and effort toward relevant activities
2. difficult goals lead to greater effort
3. goals increase persistence, with difficult goals prolonging effort (so long as they are not too difficult, which may lead to apathy)

4. goals indirectly lead to the discovery and use of task-relevant knowledge and strategies

Stajkovic and his colleagues (2006) found that specific, difficult goals lead to higher performance than either easy goals or instructions to 'do your best', as long as feedback about progress is provided, the person is committed to the goal and the person has the ability and knowledge to perform the task.

Self-concordant goals

Goals that are pursued to fulfil intrinsic values or to support an individual's self-concept are called self-concordant goals. Self-concordant goals fulfil basic needs and align with an individual's 'true self'. Because these goals have personal meaning to an individual and reflect an individual's self-identity, self-concordant goals are more likely to receive sustained effort over time (Gollwitzer 1990). A goal that is imposed on a student by a teacher or parent is not a self-concordant goal.

Furthermore, self-determination theory shows that if an individual effectively achieves a goal, but that goal is not self-concordant, wellbeing levels do not change despite goal attainment (Ryan & Deci 2000).

Having personal goals that are selected for autonomous reasons increases goal-directed effort and thereby increases goal progress. Goal progress, in turn, leads to an increase in subjective wellbeing and adjustment (Vasalampi et al 2009).

Mastery goals

Focus on process, not product

In order for students to achieve their goals, they must be process-focused, not product focused. In particular, they must begin to value a journey of slow growth, rather than getting to a destination quickly. The desire to achieve results quickly fools us into thinking that the result is the prize, when in reality it is the working towards something of value that enhances our lives.

Too often, after people have achieved a goal (for example – to lose eight kilograms), they will revert to old ways of thinking and doing. This reverting back leads them to undo their good work and the result they had worked so hard for. This creates a 'yo-yo' effect.

A better goal may be to consider the sort of person we want to be. That is, we might want to be a healthy person, or someone who exercises four or five times a week. This is not a destination goal; rather it is a process goal. It is a matter of continually doing the actions that lead to the desired results. Focusing on a process is a great way to keep a scorecard of our goals, as well as to continue the journey beyond the realisation of a goal.

Focus on practice, not performance

Another way to think about this is to focus on the practice, rather than on the performance. For example, if a sports team wants to win a grand final, they should focus on what they do at practice each session. If an adult wants to lose weight, they should focus on their daily nutrition and exercise program. If students want to achieve academic success, they should focus on improving the quality and regularity of their study. If we focus on the process, the performance takes care of itself.

In each of these examples, focusing on the process allows for improvement and makes the achievement of the goal possible. After the goal has been attained, in most cases real learners and improvers want to build on that accomplishment. If we don't hold on too tightly to the need for immediate results, we can continue on a growth journey for the long-term.

The importance of goals

Goals are great for prompting us to take action towards a desired future state. Your goal is like a compass that gives you direction, rather than a destination with buried treasure. Goals can also be likened to the rudder on a boat, while the actions we take (or the process) are like the engine. While the rudder (the goal) is essential for setting the direction, it is the engine (the process of making relevant daily actions) that moves the boat forward.

Target, Obstacle, Plan – T.O.P.

"How many of us start something new, full of excitement and good intentions, and then give up- permanently- when we encounter the first real obstacle, the first long plateau in progress?"
Angela Duckworth

Adolescents can struggle with setting or striving for goals that require a great deal of persistence. In fact, we all can. While schools often invite students to 'dream big dreams', 'shoot for the moon' and 'think positive', rarely does this seem to be reflected in student outcomes.

If it were easy to achieve our goals, we would already have done it. Inevitably, after we set a goal, life throws us a curveball.

Because of this reality, typical goal setting will not work in this context. However, projecting towards a desired future state, expecting setbacks along the way and creating a plan for continuing towards a goal is much more effective. Mental contrasting and implementation intentions have been found to enhance this process.

Mental contrasting

Mental contrasting is the process of contrasting our desired future state (the goal), with the obstacles that may stand in the way. Mental contrasting enhances the goal setting stage and strengthens goal commitment. While setting goals and committing to them does not turn them into a reality, the process of mental contrasting has been found to energise individuals into taking action (Oettingen et al 2009).

Implementation intentions

Once goals are set, we must then strive for them. While goal setting is enhanced through mental contrasting, goal striving is enhanced by forming implementation intentions. Essentially, this process requires making 'if/then' plans and has been shown to enhance our ability to get started or stay on track with the actions required to bring goals to fruition (Gollwitzer 1999). This plan can detail when, where and how the individual will take action.

In a study of students preparing for a high stakes exam used to determine merit-based scholarships, those students who were taught mental contrasting and implementation intentions completed over 60 percent more practice questions than students in the control condition (Duckworth et al 2011).

Rather than 'shoot for the moon', mental contrasting and implementation intentions has proven results. There are some very good support materials available for this. One such tool is an app called WOOP (wish, outcome, obstacle, plan), which is based on 20 years of scientific research by creator Gabriele Oettingen (Oettingen et al 2009). At UPP, we have simplified this process (we call it T.O.P.) to make it more accessible for all people.

Effective goal setting with T.O.P.

So, for effective goal setting we can use the three steps of T.O.P.:

1. Set a *Target* (for those familiar with S.M.A.R.T. goals, the Target should be Specific, Measurable, Time-framed, etc). It should be stated in this format: "My target is ..."
2. Think of an *Obstacle* that might get in the way.
3. *Plan* what you can do to overcome the obstacle. "If ... (obstacle happens), then ... (I will do my plan)."

Example of T.O.P. process for a high school student:

TARGET	"My target is to do 30 minutes of study before dinner every school night in term 1."
OBSTACLE	"One obstacle to doing my study is that social media can often distract me from my study."
PLAN	"If I am tempted to check out social media on my phone, then I will put my phone in a different room until I have finished my study and reward myself with checking my phone once I have finished."

By following the T.O.P. process, we are more likely to stick with the actions required to bring about our goals, when inevitable obstacles appear in our lives. We have a plan and we know exactly what we are to do when the obstacle arises.

Password goals

A useful way to fast track our goals is to create a goal orientated password to unlock our devices. We unlock our devices several times each day, therefore it is a way to be frequently reminded of our goals. Setting a password goal reminds us of what we are striving for, bringing our top priority goal into focus every time we unlock our devices.

I recently asked a group of year 11 students on a high performance camp how many of them tend to forget some of their learning goals or give up on them. Most of the group raised their hands. Then I asked how many of them would tend to open up a device (laptop/tablet/PC/phone) more than five times a day. Every single one of them raised their hand. I then proposed they set a password goal – so they will be reminded of the goal many times each day.

This seemingly small act, repeated over and over, can go a long way toward helping us stay on task with achieving our goals. By changing our passwords to reinforce a goal we are trying to accomplish, we will put it top of mind and unconsciously focus in on ways to make those things happen (Adams-Miller 2017).

Hope theory – will and way

Hope is "a feeling of expectation and desire for a particular thing to happen" (Oxford Dictionary 2018). Snyder and his colleagues argue that hopeful people believe in their ability, are able to establish clear goals, imagine multiple workable pathways toward those goals and persevere when obstacles get in their way (Snyder, Rand & Sigmon 2002).

Hope theory is comprised of:
- Goals – Approaching life in a goal-oriented way.
- Pathways – Finding different ways to achieve your goals.
- Agency – Believing that you can instigate change and achieve these goals.

(Snyder, Rand & Sigmon 2002).

It has also been referred to as having "the will and the way." Hope has been linked to higher academic performance, athletic performance, physical health and mental wellbeing.

Schools can help students develop pathways and agency thinking. "Pathways can be developed by helping students develop skills in planning, time allocation, breaking down big goals into little steps, and brainstorming numerous paths towards their goals. Agency can be developed through working in teams, using goals that are progressively more challenging, and paying attention to negative self talk that may undermine motivation." (Norrish, Robinson & Williams 2011).

Achieving more – growth mindset

"Picture your brain forming new connections as you meet the challenge and learn." – Carol Dweck

"I don't divide the world into the weak and the strong, the successes and the failures. I divide the world into the learners and the non-learners." – Benjamin Barber.

"The measure of intelligence is the ability to change." Albert Einstein

The main inhibitors to thriving, that I detailed in my first book entitled Thrive- Unlocking the truth about student performance, all reside in the mind.

Cultivating a growth mindset is the foundation for students being able to thrive in their learning and life. Are intelligence and talent things you are born with, or can they be developed over time? The answer is not one or the other.

We are born with certain predispositions. However, much of our success has to do with our life experiences. Why does Australia usually achieve poor results on the world scale in events like skiing or ice hockey but do well in sports like cricket and swimming? Why do Canadian kids born in the second half of the year have far less chance of ever making it as professional ice hockey players than their peers born in the first half of the year? How can one street in England (Silverdale Road, Reading) produce more top class table tennis players than the rest of the country combined? As a society, we tend to attribute success and accomplishments to natural talent and abilities. But this is not the whole picture. Talents and abilities are, indeed, developed over time.

Talent and ability – fixed or malleable?

Carol Dweck's research (2006) has identified two ways to explain achievement. First, that talent and ability are inherent (a fixed mindset). Secondly, that talent and ability are malleable (a growth mindset). The trouble with believing in the fixed mindset is that it severely limits our potential. With a fixed mindset, we believe we cannot change our innate abilities – so we tend not to do the work to change.

The growth mindset allows us to unleash the potential we have by applying our effort and energy to develop our abilities and talents. With a growth mindset, we can take charge of how we invest our energy and effort in our lives. William James wrote that we possess enormous "amounts of resource, which only exceptional individuals push to the extremes of use" (James 1890). The high achievers in society, and in our schools, are those who stretch their abilities further than others. It's not necessarily the case that the have more ability, just that they stretch a little further.

These beliefs are supported by research in the discipline of neuroscience. When students are taught that talent is malleable, their grades improve. If they are taught that intelligence and talent are developed over time, through focused effort and attention, they are able to let go of restrictive beliefs more easily and improve their academic outcomes (Good, Aronson & Inzlicht 2003).

Fixed or growth mindsets are created through praise, feedback and stories or articles that move students towards a particular mindset, or along a mindset continuum (Anderson, 2017). We can focus our efforts on teaching students that the brain is like a muscle that gets stronger with use and that every time students work hard and learn new things, the neurons in their brains form new connections (Dweck 2009). If we are hoping to cultivate thriving students, we will be intentional about the messages we give them.

A number of our PWP's focus on developing a growth mindset, while UPP grwoth mindset incursions focus on the concept of neuroplasticity and the amazing learning equipment that students possess (their brain) in a relevant, practical and engaging way.

Grit

> *"The only thing that I see that is distinctly different about me is I'm not afraid to die on a treadmill. I will not be outworked, period. You might have more talent than me, you might be smarter than me, you might be sexier than me, you might be all of those things – you got it on me in nine categories. But if we get on the treadmill together, there's two things: You're getting off first, or I'm going to die. It's really that simple..."* – Will Smith

> *"When the going gets tough, the tough get going."* – Joseph Kennedy

Angela Duckworth is the preeminent researcher in the field of grit. She defines it as "perseverance and passion for long-term goals" (Duckworth 2007). Grit is about determination, resolve, resilience, discipline, self-control, persistence and a willingness to do whatever it takes to achieve important goals. It is a combination of resilience and persistence.

People who are gritty are more resilient in the face of adversity, they bounce back after failure and disappointment and they persist when progress is slow, boring, tedious or difficult. Grit is a factor of both nature and nurture. We are all born different, so some of us may have a predisposition to certain character strengths – of which grit is one. Our character strengths can be further developed, based on our actions, thoughts, choices and life experience. Grit is an action, whereas growth mindset is an understanding. Grit is the action that leads to learning, improving and thriving. Growth mindset and grit are a powerful combination.

As educators, we have all encountered latent potential in the children we teach. We have seen it dormant inside them or wasted altogether. If only they could direct their energy, attention and effort into something that would help them learn, improve or grow, then their future might be different. Grit is the key to action that unlocks human potential in every endeavour. So let's get serious about equipping every kid in every school with grit.

Grit – sticking with it to the end

Grit does not simply require believing or wanting to achieve something. This is just the start of the process. A belief system and motivation are necessary but are not sufficient for the achievement of goals. Grit involves sticking with commitments until they come to fruition. It is not just about setting goals, it is about doing the things that will lead to their achievement. Grit is not about having good intentions or starting an activity – anyone can do that. Grit is about sticking with it until it is complete. Gritty individuals are distinguished by their propensity to maintain "effort and interest over years, despite failure, adversity and plateaus in progress" (Duckworth 2007).

Grit is one of the best predictors of our success in work, life and learning. It is not just about encouraging students to work harder or to be grittier. We can assist our students more by helping them to set meaningful goals for themselves, to remove distractions from their environment (this is called choice architecture) and to set up good habits (refer to Section 8 – Healthy Habits).

Practices to build accomplishment

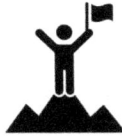

Accomplishment

ACCOMPLISHMENT	
Phone a friend	When you are stuck on a problem and you can't find a way, consider "Who could I ask for help who has been down this road before?" Then pick up the phone and they might save you hours of your time (and money) as you move towards your goals.
Win the morning	Get up a few minutes earlier than usual and exercise, meditate or practise mindfulness. Don't do all of these, rather choose the one that you like the most. It feels great to start the day proactively on the right foot, rather than reactively by sleeping in, rolling over and checking the emails on your phone.

Turn off email alerts	Turn off all email alerts and app notifications etc to increase productivity and focus and allow flow to happen.
Best possible self and dream job	Spend three minutes visualising your best possible self (10 years from now) and dream job. Then write down what you imagined under the two headings. *PWP Wk 34
A gritty person	Reflect on someone in your life, or someone you know of, who you admire and who has shown grit. Share with a friend or family member, or write it down. *PWP Wk 17
Mindsets – favourite mistake	Think about or write down the mistakes you have made in your work or life in the last couple of months, that you have learned from. These are not your favourite mistakes because you made them, they are your favourites because you have learned from them. Record the lessons learned or insight gained. *PWP Wk 15

Growth mindset – neuroplasticity	Write your name or brush your teeth with your less dominant hand this week. Observe how much you improve. *PWP Wk 14
Password goals	Decide what your top priority goal is. Next, make your goal into a password – so that you remind yourself of your goal multiple times each day. *PWP Wk 4 & PWP Wk 22
Goal setting – T.O.P.	Write down your T.O.P. 1. Set a *Target*. 2. Think of an *Obstacle* that might get in the way. 3. *Plan* if/then what you can do to overcome the obstacle. *PWP Wk 3
Three hard things	Record three hard things that you have done recently. Explain what made each of them difficult. Include how you did them and what strengths you used. *PWP Wk 2
* For more information and to lead this practice with your students, go to the relevant PWP in Part 2.	

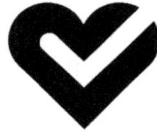

Health

Health, as defined by the World Health Organisation, is "a state of complete physical, mental and social wellbeing and not merely the absence of disease or infirmity." (WHO 2018a). Health may be defined as the ability to adapt and manage physical, mental and social challenges throughout life:

- Physical – physical and physiological health in the body and its systems
- Emotional – the presence of positive emotion and the ability to manage emotions
- Social – the presence of warm, trusting relationships and the capacity to interact with others
- Psychological – ability to handle challenges and feelings of confidence for the future (Keyes 2002, 2005).

In westernised cultures, lifestyle-related illnesses continue to be the major source of illness. Patterns of obesity, inactivity, drug use and mental health are far from encouraging and the long-term impact of these may be momentous (Hassed 2008).

We are becoming increasingly knowledgeable about the impact that thoughts and emotions can have on physiological systems, and vice versa (Libkuman et al 2007). Therefore, when you look after your body, you are also looking after your mind. And when you look after your mind, you are also looking after your body.

Being healthy involves enjoying your body when it is working well. We have all had experiences when this is not the case – for example, when you have a cold and your body does not work as well and you feel miserable. While we are all going to get sick from time to time, there are many things we can do to improve and maintain a healthy body and mind. A recent study suggests we do not 'inherit' longevity as much as previously believed. Instead, the sum of our habits determines our life span (Rath 2013).

Healthy habits

Healthy habits lead to a healthy body; this includes eating well, moving often, restful sleep and mindfully restoring our energy. These behaviours also positively support mental health, relationships and cognitive functioning. Making small, everyday choices to be healthy in what we eat, how much we move, how we sleep and how we restore our minds will lead to our overall flourishing. We will explore habits further in the next section.

Researchers have suggested that if we expend too much energy without sufficient recovery periods, eventually our body will burnout and break down (Loehr & Schwartz 2005). Mindfully restoring is taking a few moments to rest when we start to feel tired, stressed and restless – allowing us to recharge. Rather than pushing through, we need to have a brain break. Our mind affects how healthy our body is. This means that our thoughts, feelings, beliefs, and attitudes can positively or negatively affect our biological functioning. If we can take small moments when we feel overwhelmed during our day to just breathe and have a brain break, we will be more energised, focused and productive.

As we explore the topic of health, we will focus on the mind-body connection, stress, mental fitness and physical health.

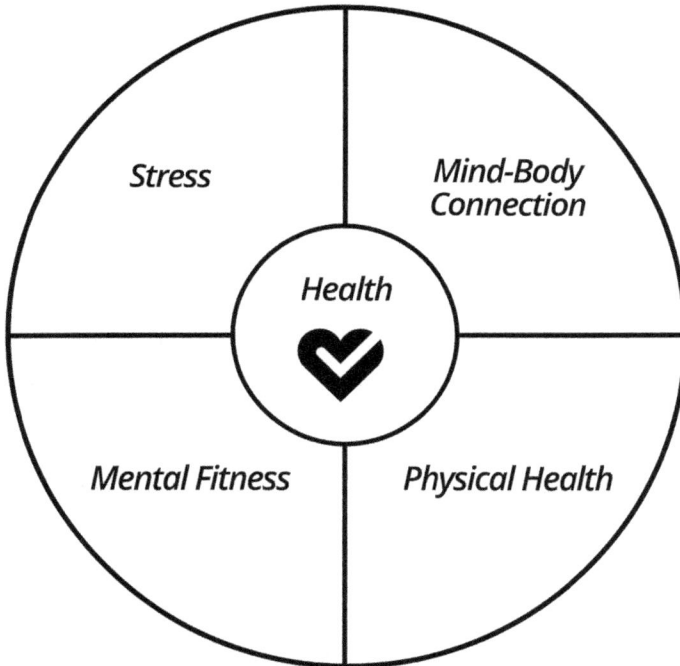

Mind-Body Connection

In the past, the mind and the body were studied separately. Recently however, there has been increased focus on holistic health, whereby the entire person is considered an integrated and interconnected entity (Hassed 2008).

Mental health has a profound and direct effect upon physical health and recovery from illness. For example, depression is a major independent risk factor for heart disease. Also, the addition of a stress management plan to cardiac rehabilitation patients nearly halves the number of ongoing cardiac events (Beyond Blue 2014). Some of the more effective programs reduce cardiac events by 74% over five-year follow-up compared to usual care alone.

Our mental and emotional state also has profound effects on our immunity and every other part of our bodies, even right down to the levels of our genes. So improving mental health is important for quality of life, to facilitate other healthy lifestyle changes, and for its direct benefits for health.

How does the mind-body connection work?

One of the key ways that the body and mind are linked can be explained by neurotransmitters. Neurotransmitters are chemicals that help us to transmit messages between neurons (Lodish et al 2000). The presence of a neurotransmitter influences the way that information is received by each subsequent neuron in a neural pathway. They play a major role in shaping everyday life and functions.

An example of this interconnectedness between the body and the mind is the fight-flight response. During a harmful, threatening or stressful situation, our brain processes the signals and releases cortisol and adrenaline (two common neurotransmitters). This then leads to other physical reactions such as increased heart rate, slowed digestion, tunnel vision, shaking and a flushed face.

While a "sequence of hormonal changes and physiological responses helps someone to fight the threat off or flee to safety, unfortunately, the body can also overreact to stressors that are not life-threatening, such as traffic jams, work pressure and family difficulties. Repeated activation of the stress response takes a toll on the body. Research suggests that chronic stress contributes to high blood pressure, promotes the formation of artery-clogging deposits, and causes brain changes that may contribute to anxiety, depression and addiction" (Harvard Medical School 2018).

Neurotransmitters

Common neurotransmitters along with their causes and functions are included below:

NAME	CAUSED BY...	FUNCTION
Dopamine	Pleasure inducing activities, exercise.	Facilitates motor control, motivation, learning, arousal, reinforcement and reward. It can give us a natural 'high' and is associated with addiction as we seek more and more dopamine.
Serotonin	Sunlight, exercise, physical contact and positive emotion.	Contributor to feelings of wellbeing and happiness, involved in emotion, mood, temperature regulation, sensory perception and wound healing.
Oxytocin (also called the 'love hormone' or the 'cuddle chemical')	Physical touch and positive social interactions (kindness, empathy, eye contact).	Responsible for social bonding, social recognition, parental care and trust building.
Melatonin	Secreted by the pineal gland in response to the daily light-dark cycle.	Regulates wakefulness, sleep cycles and possibly affects sexual development.

Endorphins	Produced in response to physical stress or pain.	Lessen the pain sensation.
Adrenaline (also called epinephrine)	Secreted by the adrenal glands in response to stress or other demands on the body.	Increases the heart rate, alertness, blood pressure and blood flow to muscles and prepares the body for dangerous and extreme situations.
Cortisol	Released from the adrenal glands as part of the body's stress response.	Suppresses the immune system, aids in the metabolism of fat, protein and carbohydrates. Prolonged exposure has damaging effects on the brain.

(Adapted from Harvard Medical School 2018; Dana Foundation 2018.)

So through our actions and life experiences, we are able to encourage or discourage the release of certain neurotransmitters. For example, to increase dopamine or serotonin, we can engage in physical activity; to increase oxytocin, we can share a hug with a loved one regularly; or, to reduce cortisol, we might practice some of UPP's PWPs in order to reduce the stress response.

While neurotransmitters can be released quickly, it is the impact of our neurotransmitters in our system over time that will determine our mind-body health. So creating healthy habits is key to good health.

Stress

Stress is a state of mental, physical or emotional tension, resulting from demanding circumstances. At different times in our lives, we all experience demanding circumstances resulting in stress – but it is not always a bad thing. There are two different types of stress – one is good or productive stress and the other is negative or distress.

Eustress and distress

A small amount of stress may be desired, beneficial and even healthy. It can sharpen our focus, as well as increase stamina and alertness to help us rise to the challenges we face.

Good stress (eustress) is when we feel uncomfortable, nervous and pressured, but believe we can handle it. It can be energising and improve our performance, and it usually only lasts a short time (Lazarus 1966). It can also inspire us to take action (finish the assignment, sort out the friendship issue). We might have this stress before an exam, or an athletic race, when meeting new people or when trying something new.

If we notice feeling stressed, we can realise that our bodies are telling us that something is important to us, and we can respond to the motivation and energy it provides. When we are able to cope with difficult and challenging situations, new learning, growth and connection will often come out as a result (McQuaid & Kern 2017).

Excessive amounts of stress, however, can lead to a prolonged 'cocktail' of adrenaline and cortisol in our brain and is potentially harmful. Distress (when a demand vastly exceeds a person's capabilities), is a threat to quality of life (Le Fevre et al 2006). It can increase the risk of strokes, heart attacks, ulcers, and mental illnesses such as depression (Sapolsky 2004). Distress can make the individual more susceptible to physical illnesses like the common cold, as it can reduce our immunity (Edmunds 1997).

We can't avoid all stress in our lives. Instead, we are better off finding ways to cope with the stressors that are bound to come our way as we journey through life. Some useful strategies for coping with stress are: mindfulness, visualisation, being organised, journaling, drawing, deep breathing, listening to relaxing music, dancing and exercise. These things have been found to reduce the stress response in our bodies. It is well worth trying a few of the suggestions outlined in our PWPs, in order to see what strategies help you the most.

There may be times when we feel that negative stress (distress) is overwhelming. At these times we should seek the support and guidance of family, trusted adult friends, school teachers or counsellors, or youth health organisations like Beyond Blue (Beyond Blue 2017), ReachOut (Reachout 2018) or Headspace (Headspace 2018).

Mental Fitness – mindfulness

"Whatever is true, whatever is noble, whatever is right, whatever is pure, whatever is lovely, whatever is admirable – if anything is excellent or praiseworthy – think about such things." – Philippians 4:8

Mindfulness is the psychological process of bringing our attention to experiences occurring in the present moment (Kabat-Zinn 2013; Creswell 2017), which we can develop through the practice of meditation and through other training (Kabat-Zinn 2013; Lutz, Davidson & Slagter 2011; Deatherage 1975). The objective is to welcome and accept the current state including any emotions, thoughts and perceptions (Kabat-Zinn 2003).

Research studies have consistently shown a positive relationship between mindfulness and psychological health (Tomlinson et al 2018; Keng, Smoski & Robins 2011). Studies also indicate that rumination and worry contribute to the onset of a variety of mental disorders (Kaplan et al 2017; Watkins 2015; Querstret & Cropley 2013) and that mindfulness-based interventions significantly reduce both rumination and worry (Querstret & Cropley 2013; Gu et al 2015; Perestelo-Perez et al 2017).

Mindfulness as prevention

Further, the practice of mindfulness may be a preventive strategy to halt the development of mental-health problems (Tang and Leve 2015; Cheng 2016). Mindfulness also seems to have a positive impact on the physical body – calming of the stress response and improving immunity (Hassed 2008). In studies of adolescents, mindfulness has been found to have a beneficial impact on physical health, mental health, social skills, focused attention and even reduce problematic school behaviours (Black, Milam & Sussman 2009; Burke 2010).

Mindfulness is about paying attention and noticing ourselves and the things around us in a particular way. Sometimes our minds wander – we just go through the motions and our minds are not focused on what we are doing in the present moment. We might eat without tasting, look without seeing and talk without really knowing what we are saying.

Mindfulness is the awareness that emerges through paying attention on purpose, in the present moment, and nonjudgmentally, to the unfolding experience (Kabat-Zinn 2003). Mindfulness is an active process leading to awareness. We focus on the present rather than the past or future and we accept what is, without labelling it good or bad.

Cultivating mindfulness leads to reduced stress and anxiety, improved sleep, greater self-awareness, less anger and frustration, increased confidence, better relationships, improved capacity for focus and concentration, better learning and greater levels of enjoyment in life (Greco et al 2005; Semple et al 2006).

Mindfulness can be practised in activities such as eating, washing hands, drawing, colouring in and walking (Dimidjian & Linehan 2003). We can simply go about our daily activities mindfully, which allows us to welcome and accept our current state, rather than focus on past disappointments or future worries (Kabat-Zinn 2003). It can also be practised through meditation.

Meditation

Meditation takes our thinking out of the past or the future and aims to bring us into the present moment. If it was a drug that we could purchase over the counter it would be a best seller – with so many benefits and no side-effects.

When I explain meditation to students, I ask them to imagine that they have a Ferrari of a mind. If they are driving around constantly in a Ferrari, they will sometimes need to refuel. They would need to park the car, put the handbrake on and add fuel, oil and brake fluid from time to time.

Our mind is rushing around constantly, thinking about the past or anticipating the future. We have so many intellectual demands and so many stimuli each day that the mind doesn't naturally get much respite. I tell students to put the hand brake on and refuel. Park the Ferrari that is their mind. It doesn't take long, it doesn't cost them anything and the benefits are supported by a huge body of evidence. For educators and parents, we should do this for our own sake. Once we do, we will want to share it with the children in our care.

Benefits of meditation

There are significant physical and psychological benefits of meditation. There is a wealth of evidence that demonstrates the effects meditation has on managing stress, combating heart disease, lowering blood pressure, boosting our immune systems, building our defence against cancer, slowing the rate at which we age, improving our mood, raising our awareness and increasing attention and clarity (Michie 2008; Davidson et al 2003). Other benefits include reducing fear, anxiety, depression and anger.

These benefits come about as a result of the adaptation of the brain over time, due to the brain activity associated with meditation. These benefits have been found to last much longer than the meditation session itself, because it changes some of the default settings in our brain (Brewer et al 2011). Meditation based interventions have been found to correlate with a significant grey matter increase (Kurth et al 2014; Holzel et al 2011; Fox et al 2014). It has been noted that both the thickness of the prefrontal cortex and the density of grey matter increase as a result of meditation (Lazar et al 2005; Davidson & Lutz 2008). These very well documented changes are collectively termed 'the relaxation response' (Benson 1997).

As with all of the PERMAH elements, learning about mindfulness is not enough. We must practise mindfulness regularly if we are to experience the benefits (Huppert & Johnson 2010). We need to 'take the medicine' for it to actually work. It doesn't work, unless we do the work.

At this point, we can look to four of the more common meditation techniques.

Breathing meditation

This meditation involves counting the breath going in and out. For example, breathing in for four counts, pausing, then breathing out for four counts. Many variations of counts can be used here. For example, breathe in for three, hold for one then breathe out for five. Personally, I think you should find a pattern that works for you and that draws your attention to your breathing without making you uncomfortable.

Body-scan meditation

A body-scan meditation usually involves a process of drawing awareness to different parts of the body, in a related sequence. It is not about trying to fix pain or tension, but rather being aware of it and accepting it. It is best taught to students lying down on their backs, with their eyes closed.

Participants draw their attention and focus to a part of the body and notice the sensations in that area, before moving on to the next area. It is a useful way of drawing the focus away from the past and future happenings in our mind and drawing ourselves into our body at the present time.

Mindfulness meditation

This meditation is centred on the idea of being mindful. Rather than following any thoughts that come into our Ferrari of a mind, we simply let them go and keep coming back to the breath. We are mindful of the air coming in through our nostrils. As we inhale, we notice that our stomach rises (much like a balloon that inflates as the air goes into it). As we exhale, the stomach falls. Students can do this meditation sitting or lying down, but they should place one or both hands on their stomach, to assist them in being aware of the rise and fall of each breath.

Loving kindness meditation (LKM)

Of all the types of meditation, loving kindness meditation has been found to have the greatest impact on increasing our positive emotions. LKM can increase love, joy, contentment, gratitude, pride, hope, interest, amusement, awe (Fredrickson et al 2008) and positive emotions (Kok et al 2013).

Through loving and kind concern for the wellbeing of ourselves and other people, it has been found to broaden attention, enhance positive emotions and reduce negative emotional states, while increasing empathy and compassion. LKM is considered particularly helpful for people who have a tendency toward hostility or anger (Analayo 2003). LKM consists of directing love and kindness "towards oneself, toward specific others or in all directions to all beings" (Hofmann, Grossman & Hinton 2011).

The method requires us to simply bring the body into stillness and focus attention on the breath. Then attention is turned towards oneself. We simply offer love and kindness to ourselves. (We might offer a statement to ourselves, such as "May I be happy, may I be at peace, and may I be held in deep compassion.") Then we offer the same to someone we hold close to our hearts. Then we offer love and kindness to someone we find difficult. The final part of the process is offering love and kindness to all human beings, including those we do not know.

Meditation summary

While each of these meditations will take an investment of time to set expectations with groups of students, the time required lessens over time. It should also be noted that each of the descriptions above is brief and simple, just to give you an idea of the process for each. Smiling Mind has a great app and some wonderful YouTube clips with age appropriate meditation techniques that teachers and parents can access for free. You will also notice some guided meditations in our PWPs.

The benefits of meditation are significant and well-researched. It is as useful for adults as it is to children, and it can be taught with little time. In fact, I would suggest that two minutes of meditation at the start, or at the halfway point, of a lesson, actually increases total time on task during the lesson. In addition, it will increase the quality of work, the attention and focus of the students and lead to greater wellbeing.

Physical Health – move, sleep, eat
a) MOVE

> *"Physical fitness is not only one of the most important keys to a healthy body, it is the basis of dynamic and creative intellectual activity."* – John F. Kennedy

More energy

If we eat, move and sleep well today, we will have more energy tomorrow (Rath 2013). When we are being active – whether walking to school, playing sport, jumping, climbing a tree, doing a dance or anything that gets our heart and lungs working, we are building a healthy body and mind. We are giving our bodies more strength, stamina, flexibility, balance and coordination.

Healthy mind

Being active also improves our concentration, self-confidence and thinking skills. Exercise enhances the way our brain works by releasing neurotransmitters such as serotonin, dopamine and adrenaline, and it increases the levels of brain chemicals (called growth factors). All of these chemicals help to make new brain cells and establish new neural connections – leading to improved learning, memory and attention (McQuaid & Kern 2017).

Regular exercise is also an important part of maintaining good mental health for everyone, whether old or young, for example, in helping to raise self-esteem and prevent or treat depression (Dunn et al 2005) and anxiety (Byrne & Byrne 1993).

Physical health

Exercise has been shown to be restorative (Bauman 2004). Being active every day keeps us healthy and helps prevents illness. Lack of exercise is the second highest cause of disability and death in Australia (after smoking) (AIHW 2001). People who exercise regularly are less likely to die from heart disease (Maiorana et al 2000; Berlin & Colditz 1990; Tanasescu et al 2002) as a result of improvements in blood pressure and reduction in insulin resistance.

Regular exercise also helps prevent many cancers, including colon, breast, lung and possibly prostate cancer and other conditions such as diabetes and osteoporosis. It has even been shown that if a person contracts cancer, regular exercise makes them less likely to die from it (Colditz, Cannuscio & Grazier 1997; Thune & Lund 1997; Friedenreich et al 2004).

b) SLEEP

> *"Take care of your body. It's the only place you have to live."*
> – Jim Rohn

Restful sleep, being active and eating healthily are all connected to each other. When we get a good sleep at night, it makes it easier for us to eat well and move more the next day. These things have a flow on effect and can cause either an upward or downward spiral in our daily lives.

Research has shown exercise can help to improve not only the quantity of sleep but also the quality: daytime physical activity can stimulate longer periods of slow-wave sleep, the deepest and most restorative stages of sleep (Breus 2013). Getting enough sleep is really important, as during sleep our body repairs itself, while our mind is able to rest and consolidate previous learning.

We all have a natural sleep and waking cycle – if we disrupt this cycle, we can find it hard to get to sleep. It can also make us irritable and lead to low concentration and health issues such as heart problems, weight gain and depression. Having a bedtime routine is a great way to cue our bodies for rest (Rath 2013). This might include journaling, listening to quiet music, reading, prayer, doing some gentle yoga or meditation.

To help maintain our natural rhythm we should turn off electronics a few hours before sleep, at roughly the same time every night. The exposure to light from our devices suppresses melatonin (our sleepy neurotransmitter), making it harder to fall asleep and decreasing sleep quality.

c) EAT

"Every time we eat is an opportunity to nourish our bodies."
Author unknown

Food is a powerful medicine (Hassed 2008). We are what we eat, and we need food as fuel for our bodies. Everything we eat has a short and long-term health effect on our bodies. The food choices we make affect our health, mood, energy and physical appearance. Food is the source of energy for all parts of our bodies and directly affects how our body and mind work.

It is well known that a balanced diet consists of plant foods, such as vegetables and fruit, grain-based foods as well as moderate amounts of animal foods, such as lean meat and dairy products. Most people in western societies have a huge choice of what they will eat, but we don't always choose well.

Faced with the choice of an extra serve of vegetables or saving room for dessert ... which one would you choose? Probably not the steamed cabbage!

Sugar

Sugar-laden foods such as desserts, chocolate and carbonated drinks provide us with a fast source of energy. Apart from the calories we are consuming however, what is all this sugar doing to our brain?

Sugar stimulates the brain by releasing dopamine, which creates a natural high and prompts us to crave more. Too much sugar has an effect on the brain that is similar to cocaine and other addictive drugs (Barclay 2014). This may be why we crave chocolate or ice-cream when we're stressed, rather than broccoli!

Fats and oils

And what about excess fats and oils? In 2004, a study by Hakkarainen and his associates examined the impact of diets on the mental health of 29,133 older male smokers, who recorded their daily meals. Results showed that higher intake of processed foods with high levels of saturated fats was linked to increased anxiety, depression and insomnia. If you've seen the movie 'Fast Food Nation', you'll have seen convincing evidence of the harm that can come about by eating nothing but McDonald's for 30 days!

Water

Drinking water is also extremely important for our bodies – not having enough fluid in our body can cause headaches, fatigue, make us feel cranky and affect our concentration. Water helps keep our body temperature stable, it carries nutrients and oxygen to our cells, cushions joints, protects organs and tissues and removes waste.

When we make healthy food and hydration choices, we are more likely to enjoy wellness in our body and mind, we will have more energy for being active, we will have better sleep as a result and the cycle will continue.

Practices to build health

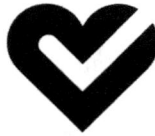

Health

HEALTH	
Stop and eat lunch	Between playground duty, classes, meetings and preparation, there is not a lot of time left over. But, make a point to step away from the desk or computer each day and eat. Even if it's only for 10 minutes.
Leave the laptop	Set boundaries on when, where and how much you work. Set a goal to not check work emails at home each night, or leave the laptop at work at least once a week.
Mindfulness strategies	Sitting quietly and comfortably, think of: • 5 things you can see; • 4 things you can touch; • 3 things you can hear; • 2 things you can smell; • 1 thing you can taste. *PWP Wk 37

Mindful walking	Take a walk slower than normal pace. With each step, be aware of the gentle heel-to-toe rhythm as each foot makes contact with the ground. Carefully notice your foot, inside your sock, inside your shoe. *PWP Wk 30
3-minute stress buster	Move your body for 1 minute, count your pulse for 1 minute as a mindful activity, deep breathe to calm your mind and body for one minute. *PWP Wk 29
Healthy habits	Think of one easy healthy food option you could have as a snack when you are hungry. Buy them from the shop and discard the unhealthy alternative that you often seek out. *PWP Wk 21
Healthy habits – sleep	Set a time to switch off all electronic devices each night. Alternatively, put an alarm on your phone to indicate when you can start your bedtime wind down routine. *PWP Wk 20
Healthy habits – let's get physical	Think of one way today that you can be a little more active. It might be as simple as parking a little further from work or getting off the bus one station early. *PWP Wk 1

Staying healthy	Practice calm or belly breathing for 10 slow, controlled breaths. As you breathe in and out, feel the stomach rise and fall. Your chest should remain still. Take 10 mindful breaths before you roll over to sleep each night. *PWP Wk 18
Mindfulness body scan	Practice a mindfulness exercise today. Either be mindful when eating, washing hands, drawing, colouring in or do a mindful body scan. *PWP Wk 9

* For more information and to lead this practice with your students, go to the relevant PWP in Part 2.

> *"We are what we repeatedly do. Excellence, then, is not an act, but a habit."* – Aristotle
>
> *"Sow a thought and you reap an action, sow an action and you reap a habit, sow a habit and you reap a character, sow a character and you reap a destiny."* – Ralph Waldo Emerson
>
> *"Chains of habit are too light to be felt until they are too heavy to be broken."* – Warren Buffett

In order to build our capacity in any of the PERMAH elements, we need to take action. The challenge is that when we start something, it is easy to fall back into our old ways. In order to help us implement the actions we want to take, we can look to build some habits for wellbeing. So let's explore how habits work.

How habits work

New behaviours can become automatic through the process of habit formation. Old habits are hard to break and new habits are hard to form because the behavioural patterns which humans repeat become imprinted in neural pathways. But it is possible to form new habits (Rosenthal 2011).

Automaticity is the ability to do things without occupying the mind with the low-level details required, allowing it to become an automatic response pattern or habit. It is usually the result of learning, repetition and practice.

Habits are responses that are activated automatically. These responses are usually activated by cues that have occurred simultaneously with responses in the past. In Charles Duhigg's best seller 'The Power of Habit', he defines habits as "the choices all of us deliberately make at some point, and then stop thinking about but continue doing, often everyday" (Duhigg 2013).

William James once said that we are "mere bundles of habit" (James 1890). Our daily actions can have a great impact on our lives when the effect is compounded over time. A Duke University study has shown that it is "actually people's unthinking routines – or habits – that form the bedrock of everyday life. Without habits, people would be doomed to plan, consciously guide, and monitor every action" (Neal, Wood & Quinn 2006).

Neural evidence indicates that with repetition, the brain 'chunks' whole sequences of responses. Essentially, our habits form over time as repeated thoughts or actions lead to strengthening neural connections. This means that "habits require limited conscious control to proceed to completion" (Neal, Wood & Quinn 2006). The behaviour becomes automatic. By understanding this pattern and how it works, we can rebuild these patterns in any way we choose.

As Neal and his associates explain, "People often fail in their attempts at changing everyday lifestyle habits such as their diet and level of exercise. Such failures are understandable given that cues such as time of day and location trigger repetition of past responses. Failures to change do not necessarily indicate poor willpower, but instead the power of situations to trigger past responses. Habits keep us doing what we have always done" (Neal, Wood & Quinn 2006).

The value of habits

Many of the decisions we make each day are habitual. One study suggests that approximately 45 percent of our everyday actions are habits in the sense that they are performed almost daily and usually in the same location (Wood, Quinn & Kashy 2002). Habits make our lives easier as we don't need to invest a lot of energy and effort into doing them.

Habitual behaviour has been linked to reduced stress levels when compared to non-habitual behaviour. It is believed the reason for this is that less thought is necessary to guide our actions when we are behaving habitually (Wood, Quinn & Kashyal 2002). When a habit emerges, our brain stops fully participating in decision making (Duhigg 2013).

However, our brain can't tell the difference between good habits and bad ones – which means that our habits can work for us, or against us. For this reason, if we want to create positive results in our lives, "we should make our nervous system our ally, instead of our enemy" (James 1890).

In order to be gritty and achieve more success, we can form habits that work in our favour. In order to do this, we must understand the habit loop, keystone habits and that willpower isn't enough.

Habit loop

Our habits can be broken into three steps:
1. The cue or trigger: the event that starts the habit (triggers could include time of day, other people, a location, a preceding event or an emotional state).
2. The routine or behaviour: the behaviour that you perform (the habit itself).
3. The reward: the benefit that is associated with the behaviour.

When we want to begin a new habit or cease an existing one, we use the habit loop. For example, if I would like to meditate more regularly (this is step 2, the routine), I must find an appropriate trigger. For example, when I put the keys in the ignition of my car each morning (this is step 1, the trigger), I will meditate for one minute. If I would like to practise gratitude (the routine) more regularly, I should align it to an appropriate trigger. This might be brushing my teeth, getting into bed or taking off my shoes each evening. Yet another example would be linking a new desired routine (going to the gym) to a regular daily trigger (driving home from work). New habits that we create should be small and easy to follow, so that we can achieve small wins and begin to strengthen the habit loop. Example below:

CUE / TRIGGER	When I put the keys in the ignition of my car each morning
ROUTINE / BEHAVIOUR	I will meditate for one minute
REWARD	Enjoying the benefits of meditation, as well as the satisfaction of doing what I set out to do.

If we are trying to cease an existing habit, like eating less chocolate, we should identify our triggers and replace the routine. For example, if I usually get peckish about an hour after lunch each day (the trigger) and begin looking for a snack, I should instead ensure that I have a healthy snack on hand at that time of day. I will still get the same trigger, but I have replaced the existing (unhealthy) routine with something more desirable. It is far more effective to replace existing negative habits than it is to eliminate them.

Keystone habits

Some habits are strongly linked to other habits. These are called 'keystone habits'. For example, if I am able to stick to the (keystone) habit of getting up and doing some exercise, it has a flow-on effect throughout my day. Typically, after exercise my body craves good food rather than junk. It has me feeling energised, focused and more productive at work. Due to the exercise, I sleep better at night. One habit is linked to a number of others.

Someone might replace smoking with walking, and this would have a flow-on effect. The change of the keystone habit may lead to a change in diet, working, sleeping, saving money, scheduling work time, building a relationship with the person I walk with, planning for the future and so on.

Keystone habits allow us to focus our energy and attention on just a couple of areas, and the flow-on effect takes it to many other areas. For students, one keystone habit that I have noticed over the years is the regular use of the student diary. If they have a system in place for managing and recording their responsibilities and learning tasks, they tend to cope with the demands much better. This keystone habit can have a flow-on effect into all other areas of their lives. Another one is sleep. A negative keystone habit that many teachers have noticed lately is online gaming. This can lead to lack of sleep, fatigue at school, inability to focus, poor results and motivation, and so on.

You can use this knowledge in order to support your best decision making. Often it starts with getting the little things right. For students, it may involve making the bed each morning, or ensuring that their school locker is tidy, organised and structured. They can then carry this composure and organisation with them to their classes.

As parents and educators, we should consider keystone habits in our own lives. This will help us to live more fulfilling lives and to model good habits to the young people we care about. We also have the opportunity to help our children or students to identify some keystone habits in their own lives that will lead them towards fulfilment and satisfaction.

Willpower doesn't work

Self-control (or willpower) is the ability to regulate one's emotions, thoughts and behaviour in the face of temptations and impulses (DeLisi 2014; Diamond 2013). Self-control is necessary for regulating one's behaviour in order to achieve specific goals (Diamond 2013; Timpano & Schmidt 2013).

Self-control is like a muscle. According to several studies, self-regulation was proven to be a limited resource which functions like energy (DeWall et al 2007). In the short term, overuse of self-control will lead to depletion. However, in the long term, the use of self-control can strengthen and improve over time (Diamond 2013; Muraven, Baumeister & Tice n.d.).

Kelly McGonigal defines willpower as "the ability to do what you really want to do when part of you really doesn't want to do it." It consists of three competing elements:
1. I will – the ability to do what you need to do
2. I won't – the other side of self-control; the ability to resist temptation
3. I want – your true (future) want, the ability to remember the big picture of your life (McGonigal 2012).

Willpower is a resource that gets depleted, particularly when you are rundown or hungry. However, you may increase your capacity for willpower by engaging in activities such as mindfulness, meditation and exercise and/or by ensuring good nutrition and adequate sleep (McGonigal 2012).

An example of an individual who may have depleted their willpower would be a worker in times of stress. In this situation, an employee will use all of their willpower to work hard, and everything else collapses as a result. They are able to muster up the energy to get out of bed early and get to work but their diet may go downhill. They will do what they need to do, however, they will not have any extra willpower to do the things that align with their core values such as spending quality time with family, eating well or exercising. At these times, it can all seem too much. Their willpower reserves are depleted.

For teachers, end of semester reporting deadlines are a difficult time. We must appear as though we have it all under control. The reality is that we need to assess, mark and report on all of our kids – while simultaneously planning, teaching and carrying out business as usual. However, every member of the school is experiencing the same raised levels of stress (staff and students alike). Schools can be a terrifying place at this time!

In any case, during this period of assessing, reporting and continued teaching, many teachers experience depleted willpower. It requires so much of us to carry out our work responsibilities that our regular diet and exercise regimes can very easily be abandoned. In these cases, we need some strategies to compensate for our depleted willpower. Two such strategies are choice architecture and the 20-second rule.

Choice architecture

Over time, our willpower can become used up, or depleted, much like tired muscles (Baumeister & Tierney 2012). As a result, we cannot rely on willpower in order to stick to good habits.

In a study using chocolate chip cookies and unsolvable problems, participants were divided into three groups:

1. Those who could see the cookies and were allowed to eat them
2. Those who could see the cookies and were not allowed to eat them
3. Those who had no cookies in sight.

It was found that the people who were told not to eat the chocolate chip cookies in front of them gave up very easily on the subsequent unsolvable puzzles. Those who were allowed to eat the chocolate chip cookies, or who had no chocolate chip cookies in sight, lasted much longer than those who could see them and were required to use willpower to deny themselves.

In another study, it has been found that only 20 percent of dieters are able to keep off the lost weight for any extended length of time (Ansel 2009). Relying on willpower and a dose of motivation, goal setting or even a New Year's resolution does not seem to work in most cases. We need more than this – and so do the students that we teach.

We need to carefully design our default choices – making it easier to make the right decisions impulsively. "When your willpower is depleted, you are even more likely to make decisions based on the environment around you. After all, if you're feeling drained, stressed, or overwhelmed then you're not going to go through a lot of effort to cook a healthy dinner or fit in a workout. You'll grab whatever is easiest" (Clear 2014a).

Choice architecture is about designing our environment so that the easiest choice to make is a better one. For example, placing healthy foods in more visible spots in the fridge, pantry or even on the bench and moving less healthy food options out of sight.

A study at Massachusetts General Hospital aimed at helping people make better food choices by using choice architecture (Thorndike et al 2012). Simply by adding fridges filled with water, and putting water in baskets around the hospital cafeteria, customers changed their buying habits for the better. In only three months, soft drink sales dropped by 11.4 percent. Meanwhile, bottled water sales increased by 25.8 percent. People made better choices as the default choice was improved.

In order to preserve your willpower for when you need it most, you can use choice architecture. Doing so will ensure that the environment you surround yourself with will ultimately lead to positive default actions. On a cold winter morning, I would prefer to stay in bed than to get out, get dressed and go for a run. Especially if I need to search for my exercise gear in the dark, as I try not to wake up the rest of my family. However, I have found that if I put my shoes, socks and running clothes beside my bed it is much easier to throw them on and get out there. Doing so improves my default choice – this is choice architecture. I have already started the process of doing a workout the night before (by getting the clothes ready) and I simply need to finish what I started.

The 20 second rule is a very practical application of choice architecture.

The 20-second rule

Mihaly Csikszentmihalyi has coined the term 'activation energy' to describe a concept similar to inertia (Csikszentmihalyi 1997). However, instead of referring to the tendency of an object to remain at rest or moving on its current path, activation energy refers to our actions and choices which take the path of least resistance. Inactivity is the easiest option.

So, how can we use this concept to assist us in the default choices we make? It is simple – we can use what Shawn Achor refers to as the '20-second rule'. He suggests lowering the activation energy for habits you want to adopt and raising it for habits you want to avoid. "The more we can lower or even eliminate the activation energy for our desired actions, the more we enhance our ability to jump-start positive change" (Achor 2010).

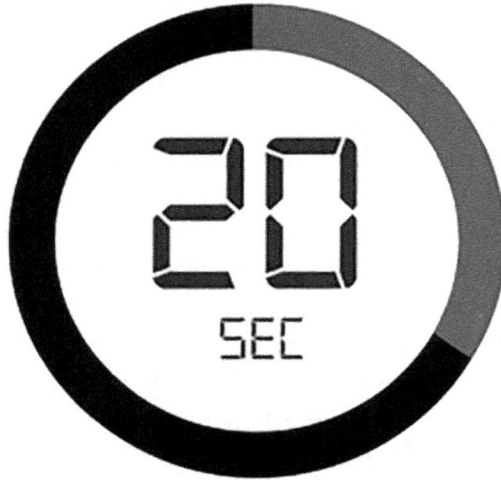

Essentially, we can ask ourselves these two questions:
How can we make it 20 seconds easier to do our most preferred actions?
How can we make it 20 seconds harder to do our least preferred actions?

If you want to watch TV less often and read more instead, put the remote control inside a drawer rather than on the coffee table – and then put a book on the coffee table. Whenever you sit on the couch ready to watch TV, your default choice now becomes reading a book. It only takes 20 seconds to get the remote out of the drawer; however, it has increased the activation energy required.

I also use this strategy by putting beer in the downstairs fridge, not in the kitchen. There are times when the activation energy required to go and get a beer to have with dinner actually means that I change my choice to water instead (as it is readily available in the kitchen). Once again, it only takes 20 seconds, but it is enough.

During work, I am tempted to check my emails regularly, which I know is not the best use of my time. This has led me to closing down my email tab after I have done my regular scheduled emailing. The extra 20 seconds it takes for me to open and load Gmail is a wonderful deterrent to me and helps me stay on track with my work. It has been particularly helpful for me in the writing of this book.

Having some fresh fruit on the bench in a fruit bowl, rather than in the crisper in the fridge, reduces the activation energy required to make a good choice of snack. Combine that with making unhealthy snacks harder to access (or getting rid of them altogether) and it becomes much easier to make great choices.

Parents and educators can also use choice architecture in study environments, study schedules or daily routines with children and students.

Can you think of one or two ways to apply the 20 second rule in your everyday life?

Now that we have investigated each of the components of PERMAH in detail, along with building healthy habits, it's time to put what we have learned into action. In order to do this, the next part of this book will outline the Personal Wellbeing Practices that we have developed for primary schools and secondary schools.

PART 2

Introduction

Part 1 of this book focused on building a solid understanding of Wellbeing, including PERMAH and habits for those wanting to expand their knowledge and lead a Wellbeing / Pastoral Care / Positive Education initiative in their school context. Part 2 is focused on implementation and action. It is recommended for all teachers of Wellbeing and Positive Education. Part 2 is intended to be used as a guide for teachers to implement in their school communities. It can also be used by Principals and leadership teams with all of their staff.

Learning about Wellbeing and Positive Education and the principles behind it will not help if we don't apply what we learn. This highlights the importance of Part 2. There will be some overlap of content from Part 1, as the rationale provided in each PWP is intended to give teachers a basic understanding of the value or reasoning behind each of the practices. This is likely to be more than enough information for teachers of Wellbeing/Positive Education or individuals wanting to take action to improve their own wellbeing. However, those who would like to learn more should be encouraged to read and study Part 1.

2.1 Personal Wellbeing Practices

What is a Personal Wellbeing Practice?

A Personal Wellbeing Practice (PWP) is an evidenced-based positive psychology intervention, applied in school communities or other educational settings. At UPP, we have tried to make these PWPs simple, concise and relevant for students and their teachers. The PWP details in this next section have been created for Secondary schools. Primary school educators should refer to Part 2.2 of this book for PWPs of a suitable level (although many of the PWPs provided in this section have been adapted successfully by primary school teachers), while Parts 2.3 - 2.6 are relevant for both primary and secondary contexts.

We have 40 PWPs available online. They are primarily related to one of the PERMAH elements. However, you will certainly notice that many of the PWPs will cross over more than one of the elements.

How are the PWPs designed to work in your school?

- We have created a guide for schools, including a rationale and an activity for teachers to implement with class groups of students in less than 10 minutes each week. Each activity requires very little equipment. If more than a pen and paper is required, this is indicated before the rationale.
- These PWPs are ready to be implemented in classrooms at your school. Each PWP will focus on one (or more) of the PERMAH elements, and they have been designed to suit the

natural ebb and flow of school life in the typical 10-week term.

- While some schools choose to implement a whole school approach, others engage a focus group, such as a year level. In either case, it is vital that teachers understand the value of the process for their students (in terms of moving towards personal and community thriving and the other positive impacts that are associated with positive mental health).

- At UPP, we offer a workshop for students entitled "An Introduction to Wellbeing with PERMAH". This is the best way that we have found to introduce students to these topics-ensuring engagement for all students and consistency of delivery to the whole year level. It also is helpful for launching such an initiative, because it helps to get the "buy-in" of students and teachers. However, having an UPP workshop is not a prerequisite for doing the PWPs.

Our hope for PWPs

We hope that allowing schools access to these evidence-based tools of positive psychology will help people to thrive and live their best life, both within and beyond the school gates. We hope to equip people (young and old) with a wellbeing toolkit that they can use regularly.

UPP's PERSONAL WELLBEING PRACTICES- LISTED BY TOPIC

POSITIVE EMOTION	ENGAGEMENT	RELATION SHIPS	MEANING	ACCOMPLISH MENT	HEALTH
One nice email (Staff PWP's)	Find a way to play (Staff PWP's)	Offer micro moves (Staff PWP's)	Volunteer yard duty (Staff PWP's)	Phone a friend (Staff PWP's)	Stop and eat lunch (Staff PWP's)
Broaden and Build Brainstorm- Wk 32	Strengths Reflection (Staff PWP's)	Do a 5 minute favour (Staff PWP's)	For the sake of what? (Staff PWP's)	Win the morning (Staff PWP's)	Leave the laptop (Staff PWP's)
Happy Memory Building- Wk 35	Stand up regularly (Staff PWP's)	Forgiveness- Wk 39	Get spiritual (Staff PWP's)	Turn off email alerts (Staff PWP's)	Mindfullness Strategies Wk 37
Overcoming Negativity Bias- Wk 33	Take a strengths pause (Staff PWP's)	Kindness Catching- Wk 38	Be awed by nature (Staff PWP's)	Best Possible Self and Dream Job- Wk 34	Mindful Walking- Wk 30
Sharing our grateful moments- Wk 28	Your Superhero Strengths- Wk 36	Active Constructive Responding- Wk 13	Awe Inspiring- Wk 25	A Gritty Person- Wk 17	3 Minute Stress Buster- Wk 29
Gratitude Letter- Wk 27	Savouring the moment- Week 31	Shout outs!- Wk 12 & Wk 40	Live your Legacy- Wk 24	Mindsets- Favourite mistake- Wk 15	Healthy Habits - Nutrition- Wk 21
Laugh out Loud- Wk 26	Intrinsic Motivation- Wk 16	Act of kindness- Wk 11	Make the mundane meaningful- Wk 23	Growth Mindset - Neuroplasticity- Wk 14	Healthy Habits - Sleep- Wk 20
Attitude of Gratitude- What went well- Wk7	Me at my best- Wk 10			Password Goals- Wk 4 & Wk 22	Let's get physical- Wk 19
Sharing hope- Wk 6	Flow activity- Wk 8			Goal Setting- T.O.P.- Wk 3	Staying Healthy- Wk 18
Happy Hits- Wk 5				3 hard things- Wk 2	Mindfulness body scan- Wk 9

WEEK 1 – PERMAH Introduction – Six Elements

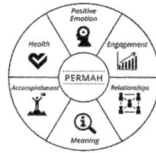

Rationale

In order to increase our wellbeing, which is our ability to do well and feel good, we are using Seligman's PERMA framework (with the added H for Health).

This research-based framework has six headings:
- **Positive emotions:** experiencing good feelings like happiness, peace and joy.
- **Engagement:** being fully involved in a task and living with interest and curiosity.
- **Relationships:** having solid relationships with self and others; feeling loved and connected.
- **Meaning:** having a purpose in life, feeling that our lives are worthwhile and serving a cause greater than ourselves.
- **Accomplishment:** striving for and achieving things that really matter to us.
- **Health:** establishing habits that increase physical and psychological health.

Teachers to read and facilitate the following with the class:

Description of Personal Wellbeing Practice: Six Elements

1. Reflecting on the six elements of PERMAH, consider which element you currently do well: *positive emotions, engagement, relationships, meaning, accomplishment or health.*
2. Why do you think this is your strongest element? Think of an example.
3. Turn to the person next to you and share with them what you think is your strongest PERMAH Element of wellbeing and why.

Main message:

The PERMAH framework provides evidence-based, actionable ways to build our own wellbeing. By building up each of these six elements that support our wellbeing, we are more able to thrive and live life to the full.

WEEK 2 – Introduction to Accomplishment – Three hard things

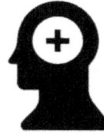

PERMAH ELEMENT

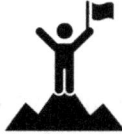

Accomplishment   *Positive Emotion*

<u>Rationale</u>

Accomplishment refers to something that has been achieved successfully. For wellbeing, this 'something' needs to matter to us. What matters is going to be different for everyone. It might mean winning an award, being proud of a task that you did, or responding in a way that makes you feel good.

Research has found that the happiest people pursue clear goals that are outside their comfort zone (Adams Miller 2017). Also, there are links between positive accomplishment, flourishing, positive emotions and wellbeing (Norrish, Robinson & Williams 2013; Sheldon et al 2010).

Basically, when we accomplish things, we feel good. When it comes to accomplishing the things that matter to you, more important than your abilities, is the belief that you can improve (McQuaid & Kern 2017). The reality is, we can all improve our current ability through effective effort.

Teachers to read and facilitate the following with the class:

Description of Personal Wellbeing Practice: Three Hard Things

When we feel like we have overcome hard things, this tends to build our self-confidence and experience of mastery. We are therefore more likely to persevere toward important goals (Adams Miller 2017).

Write down the following:
1. Record three hard things that you have done recently (e.g. started at a new school; spoke to someone in my class who I didn't know; attempted a sport I've never tried before; asked a question in class when I didn't understand).
2. Explain what made each of them difficult.
3. Include how you did them and what strengths you used.

Then, if you feel comfortable to do so, please share one of your hard things with another person in the room.

Main message:

Accomplishment involves striving for and achieving meaningful outcomes. Doing hard things that challenge you is one way to grow your abilities and confidence.

"If it doesn't challenge you, it won't change you."
– Fred Devito.

WEEK 3 – Goal Setting – Target, Obstacle, Plan – T.O.P.

PERMAH ELEMENT

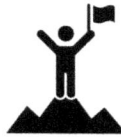

Accomplishment

Rationale

Goals give us the focus we need to direct our time, energy and effort towards things that are most valuable to us. Researchers have found that goals can provide us with motivation, help prioritise what we do and are associated with higher levels of accomplishment (McQuaid & Kern 2017).

Setting the goal is easier than following through, especially when things get hard or obstacles arise. If there were no obstacles, most people would have already achieved their targets. However, obstacles do not need to keep us from moving forward. Instead, we can use T.O.P. to overcome our obstacles. This process has been shown to enhance our ability to stay on track (by up to 60%) with the actions required to bring goals to fruition (Gollwitzer 1999).

So, for effective goal setting we can use the three steps of T.O.P.
1. Set a *Target* (For those familiar with S.M.A.R.T. goals, the Target should be Specific, Measurable, Time-framed, etc)
2. Think of an *Obstacle* that is likely to get in your way as you move towards your target.
3. *Plan* what you can do to overcome the obstacle when it arises.

Teachers to read and facilitate the following with the class:

Description of Personal Wellbeing Practice: T.O.P.

1. **Target** – Choose a target/goal that focuses on learning and growth. Then write it down, starting with "My learning target is …" E.g. "My learning target is to do 30 minutes of study before dinner every school night in term 1."
2. **Obstacle** – Next, write down one obstacle that might get in the way of your target. E.g. "One obstacle to doing my study is that social media can often distract me from my study."
3. **Plan** – Write down "If … (obstacle happens), then … (I will do my plan). Make a plan to overcome the obstacle and write it down. e.g. "If I am tempted to check out social media, then I will put my phone in a different room until I have finished my study and reward myself with checking my phone once I have finished."

Main message:

"Without goals, and plans to reach them, you are like a ship that has set sail with no destination." – Fitzhugh Dodson

WEEK 4 – Password Goals

PERMAH ELEMENT

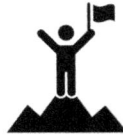

Accomplishment

Equipment required (optional)

Laptop, tablet, mobile phone or computer to use to set passwords.

Rationale

Research in the fields of neuroscience and psychology shows that goal setting actually works. The most successful people in the world set goals. A useful way to fast track our goals is to create a goal orientated password to unlock our devices. We tend to unlock our devices several times each day. Therefore, setting a password goal frequently reminds us of what we are striving for, bringing our top priority goal into focus, every time we unlock our devices.

This works because of our RAS (Reticular Activating System) in our brains. Our RAS acts as a filter for our brain – it blocks out most of the data that our brain receives every second. This allows us to increase our awareness of the things that are most important to us. By changing all of our passwords to reinforce a goal we are trying to accomplish, we will put it top of mind and unconsciously focus on ways to make those things happen (Adams Miller 2017).

Teachers to read and facilitate the following with the class:

Description of Personal Wellbeing Practice: Password goals

1. Decide what your top priority goal is. (It could be to do with school work; relationships, extracurricular, etc.) You may like to use your Target from last week's T.O.P. practice.
2. Next, make your goal password-ready. Be creative. Use shorthand, abbreviations, numbers. For example, if you want to achieve certain grades (3As and 2Bs in Semester 1), it could be 3A2Bsem1; or if you want to run 4km in 19 minutes (at the cross-country carnival this year), the password goal could be 4k19mins. Other examples are: try1newthing2day, Read20mins, 20pushups, 1actofkindness.
3. If you have access to a device, take the time now to change your password. Otherwise, do this later today.

Main message:

Fast track your goal by bringing it to top of mind with a password goal.

WEEK 5 – Positive Emotion Introduction – Happy Hits

PERMAH ELEMENT

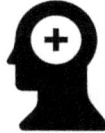

Positive Emotion

Rationale

Experiencing positive emotions like joy, gratitude, interest, hope, pride, amusement, inspiration and love has been found to benefit mental and physical health, social relationships and academic outcomes (Lyubomirsky et al 2005). Studies have shown that positive emotions help us broaden and build the way our brain responds to opportunities and challenges. This leads to us becoming more open to possibilities, connecting with others and building our resilience and wellbeing (McQuaid & Kern 2017).

Professor Fredrickson from the University of North Carolina found that when you are in a positive mood, your peripheral vision expands up to 60%. Also, we can think more quickly and creatively due to the enhanced neural connections caused by the release of dopamine and serotonin (these are neurochemicals that help our body function at its best.)

Furthermore, positivity broadens social responses and we can connect and attune better to others that can broaden and build our psychological resources. Our wellbeing is greatly enhanced from infusing more positive emotions in our lives.

Teachers to read and facilitate the following with the class:

Description of Personal Wellbeing Practice: Happy Hits

1. Write down three happy thoughts – things that bring a smile to your face. For example: a favourite song, a great memory, a funny YouTube clip you've seen, a person who makes you smile, a place that brings you peace, a funny scene from a movie. These are your 'Happy Hits'.
2. (Optional step - teacher to decide) Share this with your elbow partner (the person beside one of your elbows)!
3. Place the Happy Hits in your pocket and read them a few times during the day. Observe how your brain responds and how your mood changes throughout the day.
4. Make sure you take them out of your pocket before your clothes go through the wash! Then you can reflect on them again at home.

Main message:

Experiencing positive emotion creates an upward spiral of wellbeing.

WEEK 6 – Sharing Hope

PERMAH ELEMENT

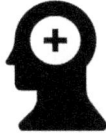

Positive Emotion   *Relationships*

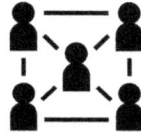

Rationale

Positive emotions help us think better and be more creative. They can undo negative emotions, make us more resilient and help us build new skills. When we look towards the future with hope, we experience the effects of the positive emotion in the present moment. Our positive emotions and experiences are deepened and our wellbeing enhanced when we share our positive experiences with someone else (Bryant & Veroff 2006).

Teachers to read and facilitate the following with the class:

Description of Personal Wellbeing Practice: Sharing Hope

1. Spend a few moments thinking about one thing you are really looking forward to in the next month. Ask yourself why you are looking forward to it.
2. Turn to the person next to you and take turns to share what you are looking forward to and why.
3. Finally, tell this person what feelings you experienced as you shared and listened.

Main message:

"Looking forward to things is half the pleasure of them. You may not get the things themselves; but nothing can prevent you from having the fun of looking forward to them." – L. M. Montgomery

WEEK 7 – Attitude of Gratitude – What went well

PERMAH ELEMENT

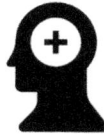

Positive Emotion

Rationale

Studies suggest that when we are grateful, we can be more optimistic, successful and healthier. Gratitude is regarded by some researchers as a "mega strategy for happiness" (McQuaid & Kern 2017). Gratitude has two parts. First, an affirmation of goodness – we notice and appreciate that there are good things in our lives and in the world. Second, discovering that the goodness comes from outside ourselves – we acknowledge that others have helped and supported us in big or small ways. One of the best ways to cultivate more gratitude is to intentionally notice and appreciate what is working well in our lives.

Teachers to read and facilitate the following with the class:

Description of Personal Wellbeing Practice: What went well

1. Think about three things that went well in the past week. They can be small, but should be things for which you feel grateful. It might have been a yummy meal, time spent doing something you love, playing a game, having a joke with a friend, something you observed in nature.

2. Write down the three things that went well.

3. Now, beside each thing that went well, write down what made these things possible. e.g. having a joke with my friend – my good friend and I have a similar sense of humour. e.g. yummy meal – because my mum decided to cook my favourite pasta dish for me last night.

Main message:

Expressing gratitude has been proven to help strengthen relationships, improve our physical health and create more positive emotions (Emmons 2010).

WEEK 8 – Engagement Introduction – Flow activity

PERMAH ELEMENT

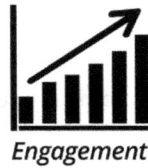

Engagement

Rationale

Flow is the peak experience of engagement – it is the feeling of being "in the zone", or *"fully immersed in a feeling of energized focus, full involvement, and enjoyment in the process of the activity"* (Csikszentmihalyi 2013). In a flow state, we tend to have intense and focused concentration and can often lose track of time.

A flow experience causes a cascade of neurochemicals – adrenaline, dopamine, endorphins, anandamide and oxytocin – to be released into our brain (Kotler 2015). This is the most potent concoction our brain can develop – a natural high. It makes us feel good. Not only that, these experiences are performance enhancing.

Creativity has been shown to increase 500-700% in a flow state. We tend to take in information faster, link together related ideas more readily, (allowing us to synthesise at a higher level) and also to connect different ideas more readily, which improves our lateral thinking (Kotler 2015). There are three main conditions that can lead to flow: clear goals and purpose; immediate feedback; and a balance of challenge and skills (Csikszentmihalyi, Abuhamdeh & Nakamura 2005).

Teachers to read and facilitate the following with the class:

Description of Personal Wellbeing Practice:
Thumb challenge for flow

(Students to face the teacher. Teacher to demonstrate.)

1. To perform the thumb challenge, make a fist with a 'thumbs up' on one hand.
2. With your other hand, point your pointer finger directly at the raised thumb.
3. Now when I (your teacher) says 'Switch', simply reverse the position, with the pointer finger on the opposite hand now pointing at the opposite thumb. When you hear 'Switch' you alternate between these two positions. Try improving your speed and coordination at each attempt.
4. Did you experience a flow state during the activity? Discuss. Was there a clear goal and purpose (complete the activity succesfully); immediate feedback (if you got it right or not); and a balance of challenge and skills (not too easy, not too hard)?
5. As a class, brainstorm activities that could encourage a state of flow. Write these on the board.

Main message:

"Flow is an optimal state of consciousness where we feel our best and perform our best. It is total absorption in a task and total focus."
– Steven Kotler 2015

WEEK 9 – Mindfulness – Mindful body scan

PERMAH ELEMENT

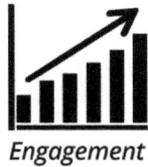

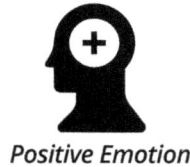

Engagement   *Positive Emotion*

Rationale

Mindfulness is about paying attention and noticing ourselves and the things around us in a particular way. Sometimes our minds wander – we just go through the motions and our minds are not focused on what we are doing in the present moment. We might eat without tasting, look without seeing and talk without really knowing what we are saying.

Mindfulness is the awareness that emerges through paying attention on purpose, in the present moment, and nonjudgmentally, to the unfolding experience (Kabat-Zinn 2003). Mindfulness is an active process leading to awareness. We focus on the present rather than the past or future, and we accept what is, without labelling it good or bad.

Cultivating mindfulness leads to reduced stress and anxiety, improved sleep, greater self-awareness, less anger and frustration, increased confidence, better relationships, improved capacity for focus and concentration, better learning and greater levels of enjoyment in life (Greco et al 2005; Semple et al 2006). Practising mindfulness involves training our minds to focus on the present moment and notice our environment, feelings, thoughts and sensations. Mindfulness can be practised in activities such as eating, washing hands, drawing, colouring in and walking (Dimidjian & Linehan 2003).

Teachers to read and facilitate the following with the class:

Description of Personal Wellbeing Practice: Mindful Body Scan

Today, we will practise a mindfulness exercise. You may choose to sit in your chair with hands in your lap, or lie down on the floor.

Before we begin, please be reminded that you should be comfortable and in your own space. You are to remain silent so as not to distract anyone else, or yourself, from the exercise.

1. Let your legs and your arms relax. Settle yourself in a comfortable position and close your eyes.
2. Start by taking two or three gentle, conscious, quiet breaths. Pay attention to how that feels. Your belly rises and falls. Air moves in and out of your body. If you like, place a hand on your belly and feel it move with each breath.
3. Now we're going to pay attention to the other parts of the body. Start with your feet. They might feel warm or cold, wet or dry, relaxed or restless. It's also okay if you feel nothing at all. If you can, relax your feet now. If that's hard to do, that's fine.
4. Now move your attention to your lower legs, noticing whatever is there. Do they feel heavy, light, warm, cold – or something else?
5. Next, move your attention to your knees and relax them. Feel the front, back and sides of your knees.
6. Notice the upper legs and let them relax. If you feel restless or wriggly, that's okay too. That happens.
7. Now move your attention to your belly. It always moves when you breathe, rising and falling, like waves on the sea. You might feel something on the inside, like full or hungry.

You might notice the touch of your clothing. You might even feel emotions in your belly, like happy or sad or upset.

8. Next, bring your attention to your chest. Notice it rising and falling as you breathe. If you feel that it's hard to focus, that's normal. Gently practise coming back again and again to how your chest feels when you breathe.

9. Now turn your attention to your hands. There is no need to move them or do anything with them. They may be touching the floor or somewhere on your body. Relax them if you can, and if not, simply pay attention to your hands for another moment.

10. Move your attention up into your arms.

11. Now move attention to your neck and shoulders, letting go and relaxing them. If your mind wanders, that's fine. Just keep returning to noticing your body whenever you find yourself thinking of something else.

12. And now feel your face and head. What expression do you have right now? What would it feel like to smile? What else do you notice in your face, your head and in your mind?

13. Finally, spend a few moments paying attention to your whole body.

14. Then open your eyes and slowly start to move or sit up.

(Adapted from Bertin 2016).

Main message:

"The best way to capture moments is to pay attention. This is how we cultivate mindfulness." – Jon Kabat-Zinn

WEEK 10 – Me at My Best

PERMAH ELEMENT

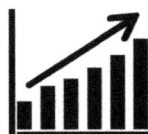

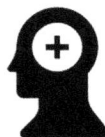

Engagement   *Positive Emotion*

Rationale

When we have the opportunity to use our strengths (the things we are good at and enjoy doing), we are more likely to feel confident, creative, satisfied and engaged (McQuaid & Lawn 2014). Strengths are ways of thinking, feeling and behaving that come naturally and easily to us and enable high functioning and performance (Linley & Harrington 2004). When we work in our strengths – in activities, relationships and learning – they energise us. They are the inner qualities that make us feel most alive and because of that, they are the areas where we have the potential to make our most meaningful contributions.

Teachers to read and facilitate the following with the class:

Description of Personal Wellbeing Practice: Me at My Best

1. Think of a time when you have been at your best (when you have been the best possible version of yourself). It might have been when you were doing something you love, or being a great friend or making a hard choice. You may have

been alone or with people. Think of how you felt and what others might have noticed.

2. Now write briefly about this time when you were at your best.
3. Finally, identify and write down what strengths you used in this situation when you were at your best.

Main message:

When we work in our strengths, we are three times more likely to report having an excellent quality of life, six times more likely to be engaged and 8% more productive (Flade, Asplen & Elliot 2015).

WEEK 11 – Introduction to Relationships – Act of kindness

PERMAH ELEMENT

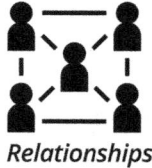

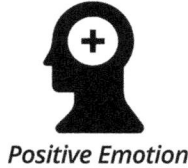

Relationships   *Positive Emotion*

Rationale

Researchers have concluded that "like food and air, we seem to need social relationships to thrive" (Diener & Biswas-Diener 2008). Our relationships with other people matter. A sense of belonging improves our self-esteem, life satisfaction and life expectancy.

We have a biological need for social support and each time we have a positive interaction with someone, our bodies release oxytocin (the pleasure inducing hormone), into our bloodstream. Oxytocin reduces our anxiety, improves concentration and helps to regulate our cardiovascular system.

We all have a psychological need to feel respected, valued and appreciated. Investing in a healthy support network is one of the best things we can do to enhance our own wellbeing. Helping and being kind to others improves our connectedness and makes us happier (Lyubomirsky 2008).

Teachers to read and facilitate the following with the class:

Description of Personal Wellbeing Practice: Act of kindness

1. Spend a few moments thinking of something good you can do for someone today (e.g. sit with someone you normally walk past at lunchtime; make afternoon tea for your sister; hold the door open for a teacher). It can be big or small but it needs to benefit them in some way.

2. Now turn to the person beside you and share what act of kindness you are going to do today. Commit to share with them next time you see them how your act of kindness made you feel and how the person responded.

Main message:

"There's no such thing as a small act of kindness. Every act creates a ripple with no logical end." – Scott Adams

WEEK 12 – Shout-outs!

PERMAH ELEMENT

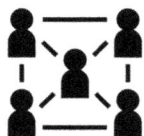

Relationships   *Positive Emotion*

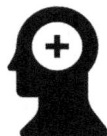

Rationale

Being kind and generous towards others is good for us. In addition to increasing our happiness and health, kindness has been found to be contagious. Researchers have found that when we receive an act of kindness, we are quite likely to 'pay it forward' (Tsvetkova & Macy 2014; Jordan et al 2013).

In essence, when we demonstrate kindness towards someone it is quite possible that the flow-on effect of our generosity will be much larger than the small act of kindness we offered. Targeted acts of kindness move us from a focus on ourselves to meeting a genuine need of someone else. They require us to be intentional and therefore are personal and meaningful. Our act of kindness this week will be through a shout-out.

Teachers to read and facilitate the following with the class:

Description of Personal Wellbeing Practice: Shout-outs!

1. Choose someone in your life who you respect or admire.
2. Think about what qualities they have that you value.

3. Write a short 'shout-out' to that person which explains these qualities. Include a specific example, if possible.
4. Share this with the person in the next 24 hours (face to face, call, email or text).

Main message:

"Wherever there is a human being, there is an opportunity for kindness." – Lucius Annaeus Seneca

WEEK 13 – Active Constructive Responding (ACR)

PERMAH ELEMENT

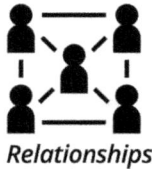

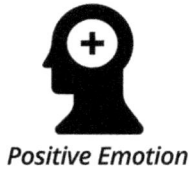

Relationships   *Positive Emotion*

Rationale

Active constructive responding (ACR) refers to the way that we respond when someone is sharing something positive with us. How we respond to the good news of others can either build a relationship or undermine it (Seligman 2011). There are four different ways of responding: active constructive (to encourage); passive constructive (to minimise); active destructive (to point out the negative); and passive destructive (to brush off or ignore).

Only one of these ways is positive for relationships – this is active constructive responding. ACR involves offering interest, enthusiasm, support, encouragement and sometimes follow-up questions when someone shares some good news with us.

An example of this might be someone sharing the good news that they are trying out for the district team. In this case, an active constructive response would be, "That is awesome! I hope the trials go well. It seems like you have been training really hard for this."

This response benefits the individual and the relationship, while the other ways of responding have been shown to have a negative impact on the wellbeing of those sharing the good news, and also on the relationship (Gable et al 2006).

Responding in an active, constructive way is a skill and can be practised to enhance relationships and wellbeing.

Teachers to read and facilitate the following with the class:

Description of Personal Wellbeing Practice: ACR

1. Turn to the person next to you so that you are in pairs. Next, we will ask a question and practise responding in an active, constructive way.
2. One person must ask their partner, "What was the best part of your last weekend?" Then listen, give eye contact and show interest in the person speaking. You can ask more questions to seek understanding and show your interest and then say something encouraging to them about what they shared.
3. Then swap so you both get a chance to listen and use active constructive responding.
4. If teachers want to practice more with the group, some other interesting questions are: What is your favourite food and why? What is your favourite book you have ever read?

Main message:

"How you respond when someone shares good news determines the quality of your relationships." – Gable, Gonzaga and Strachman

WEEK 14 – Growth Mindset – Neuroplasticity

PERMAH ELEMENT

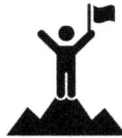

Accomplishment

Rationale

Not that long ago, it was believed that our brain's ability was fixed and set after childhood. Recently however, neuroscientists have discovered that the brain never stops changing and adjusting. Our brain is actually malleable – it can be changed and shaped through training. This process is called neuroplasticity.

Neuroplasticity is the ability of the nervous system to make large increases in the strengths of existing neural connections and also establish new connections (Pascual-Leone et al 2005). Our thoughts and actions change our brain. This means that by directing our focus, attention and action towards certain things we can strengthen our neural connections. Stronger neural connections mean that it is easier for us to do those things – like how we remember how to ride a bike.

"When it comes to learning a skill, repeated experiences are essential – as connections become stronger and more efficient through repeated use." – Nagel 2009

The plasticity of our brain allows us to improve skills through practice and repetition. For example, a right-handed person might write their name poorly with their left hand. However, through practising with the other hand, we can experience large improvements, as our neural connections strengthen. Neuroplasticity is one of the 'superpowers' of our brain – allowing us to learn many things as our brain adapts and changes.

Teachers to read and facilitate the following with the class:

Description of Personal Wellbeing Practice: Neuroplasticity

1. Today you are going to practise writing your name with your less dominant hand. Write your full name three times on a piece of paper.
2. Tonight, practice brushing your teeth with your less dominant hand for 30 seconds. Then finish brushing your teeth with your preferred hand. Continue this practice each time you brush your teeth for one week and observe how much you improve. The improvement is due to strengthening neural connections. You can strengthen neural connections for just about any skill that you choose to practise.

Main message:

"Where we make our brain go is where it will grow."
– Luke McKenna

WEEK 15 – Growth and Fixed Mindsets – My favourite mistake

PERMAH ELEMENT

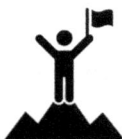

Accomplishment

Rationale

What we believe about our intelligence and talent is very important to our learning – whether we think we can grow and improve through practice, or whether think we have fixed traits that can't be improved. These beliefs are called a growth mindset or fixed mindset. A mindset can be changed.

Through the research in neuroscience we understand that we do not have a set, unchanging amount of talent. We are born with a certain amount of intelligence (albeit not very much), but through learning and effort we can improve.

People are not born walking and talking – these are skills we learn over time, as our brain adapts and our neural pathways grow. If we have a fixed mindset, we have no reason to try to improve. However, with a growth mindset we want to build and strengthen neural pathways by focusing our efforts.

When we have a growth mindset, we understand that our talents and abilities can be developed through effort, good teaching and persistence (Dweck 2006). While those with a fixed mindset tend to avoid mistakes and setbacks, those with a growth mindset understand that mistakes and setbacks are a natural part of learning – they use their mistakes to point out what they need to do to learn more and become better.

Teachers to read and facilitate the following with the class:

Description of Personal Wellbeing Practice:
My favourite mistake

1. OPTIONAL REVIEW OF LAST PWP – Discuss with one person in your class how you went over the last week attempting to brush your teeth with the opposite hand. Did you notice any improvement? What is neuroplasticity and how does it relate to brushing your teeth?
2. With a partner, share your favourite mistake of the week. While we normally don't enjoy making mistakes, 'your favourite mistake' of the week is the one that you learned the most from (e.g. You mistreated someone – and then learned that there was a better way to respond; or, you got a few answers wrong in maths – and then when you reviewed the work, you learned that you missed a step in the working.)

Main message:

"Mistakes don't make us better. Learning from mistakes makes us better."
– Luke McKenna

WEEK 16 – Motivation

PERMAH ELEMENT

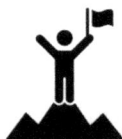

Accomplishment

Rationale

Motivation is our willingness to do something, along with the feelings that compel us to take action. Sometimes motivation comes to us when the feelings of staying the same become worse than the feelings we will get when we change our behaviour. For example, the feeling of disappointment in a test result can motivate us to work harder and spend more time studying next time. It is unlikely that we will be motivated after looking at a cute kitten poster saying 'You can do it.'

The latest research according to Daniel Pink suggests that we are either **extrinsically motivated** (having an external reward or punishment for motivation) or **intrinsically motivated** (being self-motivated).

We are most motivated in working towards the intrinsic goals of **mastery, autonomy and purpose**. i.e. mastery – the want to become a master at something; autonomy – self-direction or being able to choose; and purpose – doing something meaningful beyond ourselves. The hardest part of motivation is getting started. Once we have made even a small step towards a goal, this produces momentum that can lead to having small wins and more motivation.

Teachers to read and facilitate the following with the class:

Description of Personal Wellbeing Practice:
Exploring Intrinsic Motivation

Let's identify some instances in our lives where we have used intrinsic motivation, fuelled by purpose, autonomy and mastery. Record your answers to the following questions.

1. (Purpose) When was a time when you felt motivated to do something that was meaningful and purposeful or something that would benefit others (raising money for a good cause, helping someone who dropped an item at the shops)?
2. (Autonomy) When have you felt ownership of your work or a task and were able to choose to self-direct (chosen a topic for an assignment, chosen a sport to play at school)?
3. (Mastery) When have you been really motivated to get better at something that mattered to you (riding a skateboard, playing an instrument)?

In future, when working on tasks at school or home, it may be helpful to consider if you can connect the task to autonomy, mastery or purpose.

Main message:

"The secret to getting ahead is getting started." – Mark Twain

WEEK 17 – Getting Gritty

PERMAH ELEMENT

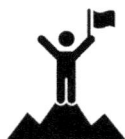

Accomplishment   *Relationships*

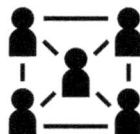

Rationale

Grit is about determination, resolve, resilience, discipline, self-control, persistence and a willingness to do whatever it takes to achieve important goals. Research leader Angela Duckworth defines grit as the combination of perseverance and passion for the pursuit of long-term goals. Enthusiasm is common but endurance is rare (Duckworth & Quinn 2009). Being gritty is hard work, but it is a key predictor of success (Duckworth 2016).

People who are gritty have the ability to stick with things until they are finished, even in the face of adversity, and they bounce back from failure or disappointment. They also persist when progress is slow, boring, tedious or difficult. Skills that contribute to grit are: delayed gratification, continuous improvement, deliberate practice, goal setting, habit formation and effort and energy management (McKenna 2015). Grit is an action that leads to learning, improving and thriving.

Teachers to read and facilitate the following with the class:

Description of Personal Wellbeing Practice – A Gritty Person

There are lots of examples of gritty people – some who are famous and others who might be your friends or family members. Parents are often very gritty as they keep working and looking after us even when they are exhausted. Our friends show that they are gritty when they persevere towards a goal – even when it is hard or they have setbacks.

At age 16, an Australian girl, Jessica Watson, attempted to sail solo and unassisted around the world. A few days before her voyage, during a test run sailing from Brisbane to Sydney, her boat, Ella's Pink Lady, collided with a 63,000-tonne bulk carrier. Watson's boat was dismasted in the collision. Many critics doubted that she could sail solo around the world. Watson had to bounce back in the face of adversity, learn from her mistake, make changes and continue to pursue her goal.

As a result of this display of grit, on May 15 2010, she became the youngest person ever to complete the seven-month, non-stop, solo circumnavigation. This is one example of a person with grit.

1. Reflect on someone in your life, or someone that you know of, whom you admire and who has shown grit.
2. Take turns in sharing with a partner about the person you admire for having grit and what you think makes them gritty.

Main message:

"When the going gets tough, the tough get going." – Joseph Kennedy

WEEK 18 – Staying Healthy – Introduction to Health

PERMAH ELEMENT

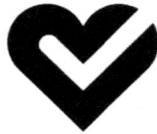

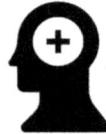

Health   *Positive Emotion*

Rationale

Being healthy involves enjoying our body when it is working well. We have all had experiences when this is not the case – for example, when we have a cold and our bodies do not work as well and we feel miserable. While we are going to get sick from time to time, there are many things we can do to improve and maintain a healthy body and mind.

A recent study suggests we do not inherit longevity as much as previously believed. Instead, the sum of our habits determines our life span (Rath 2013). Healthy habits lead to a healthy body; this includes eating well, moving often, restful sleep and mindfully restoring our energy. These behaviours also positively support mental health, relationships and cognitive functioning. Making small, everyday choices to be healthy in what we eat, how much we move, how we sleep and how we restore our minds will lead to our overall flourishing.

Researchers have suggested that if we expend too much energy without sufficient recovery periods, eventually our body will burnout and break down (Loehr & Schwartz 2005). Mindfully restoring is taking a few moments to rest when we start to feel tired, stressed and restless – allowing us to recharge. Rather than pushing through, we need to have a brain break.

Our mind affects how healthy our body is. This means that our thoughts, feelings, beliefs and attitudes can positively or negatively affect our biological functioning. If we can take small moments when we feel overwhelmed during our day to just breathe and have a brain break, we will be more energised, focused and productive.

Teachers to read and facilitate the following with the class:

Description of Personal Wellbeing Practice: Mindful breathing

1. We are going to practise calm or belly breathing. You can be seated or lying down. Before we begin, please be reminded that you should be comfortable and in your own space. You are to remain silent so as not to distract anyone else, or yourself, from the exercise.
2. Close your eyes and gently place one hand on your belly and one hand on your chest.
3. Slowly breath in through your nose, feeling your stomach rise and push against your hand. Your chest should remain still.
4. Exhale through tensed lips while tightening your abdominal muscles and feel your hand moving back down.
5. Continue to breathe for 10 breaths while focusing on feeling the rise and fall of your abdomen.

Main message:

"Feelings come and go like clouds in a windy sky. Conscious breathing is my anchor." – Thich Nhat Hanh

WEEK 19 – Let's Get Physical

Equipment required

Students will need to have some space around them to be able to do the physical movements.

PERMAH ELEMENT

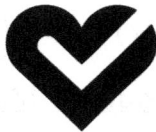

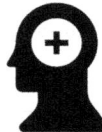

Health   *Positive Emotion*

Rationale

If we eat, move and sleep well today, we will have more energy tomorrow (Rath 2013). Being active every day is what keeps us healthy and helps prevents illness. When we are being active – either walking to school, playing sport, jumping, climbing a tree, doing a dance or something that gets our heart and lungs working, we are building a healthy body and mind. We are giving our bodies more strength, stamina, flexibility, balance and coordination.

Being active also improves our concentration, self-confidence and thinking skills. It enhances the way our brain works. Exercise releases neurotransmitters such as serotonin, dopamine and adrenaline, and increases the levels of brain chemicals (called growth factors). All of these chemicals help to make new brain cells and establish new neural connections – leading to improved learning, memory and attention (McQuaid & Kern 2017). Regular exercise is also one of the best ways to get a good night's sleep, feel good and function better.

Teachers to read and facilitate the following with the class:

Description of Personal Wellbeing Practice: Group movement

1. Each person in the class should think of a short exercise that can be done on the spot and gets your blood pumping – e.g. star jumps, running on the spot, push ups, burpees, plank, sit ups, dips, squats or an active dance move.
2. Teacher to choose five to eight students with different exercises to share with the class.
3. The whole class then completes each of the exercises for 30 seconds.

Main message:

"Physical fitness is not only one of the most important keys to a healthy body, it is the basis of dynamic and creative intellectual activity."
– John F. Kennedy

WEEK 20 – Healthy Habits – Sleep

PERMAH ELEMENT

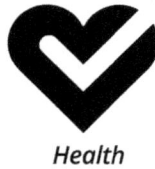

Health

Rationale

Restful sleep, being active and eating well are all connected to each other. When we get a good sleep at night, it makes it easier for us to eat well and move more the next day (Rath 2013). These things have a flow-on effect and can cause either an upward or downward spiral in our daily lives.

Research has shown exercise can help to improve not only the quantity of sleep but also the quality: daytime physical activity can stimulate longer periods of slow-wave sleep, the deepest and most restorative stages of sleep (Breus 2013).

Getting enough sleep is really important, as during sleep our body repairs itself, while our mind is able to rest and consolidate previous learning. We all have a natural sleep and waking cycle – if we disrupt this cycle, we can find it hard to get to sleep. It can also make us irritable and lead to low concentration and health issues such as heart problems, weight gain and depression. Having a bedtime routine is a great way to cue our bodies for rest (Rath 2013). This might include journaling, listening to quiet music, reading, prayer or doing some gentle yoga or meditation.

To help maintain our natural rhythm we should turn off electronics a few hours before sleep, at roughly the same time every night. The exposure to light from our devices suppresses melatonin which is our sleepy hormone, making it harder to fall asleep and decreasing sleep quality.

Teachers to read and facilitate the following with the class:

Description of Personal Wellbeing Practice: Bedtime routine

1. Think about two habits you could include in your routine to get ready for bed each night.
2. In order to implement your new bedtime routine, finish this sentence for each of your two bedtime habits.

   "I will [INSERT ACTION] every weeknight at [TIME] in [PLACE]."

   e.g. 1 – "I will [stop using my electronic devices] every weeknight at [7:30pm] in [my bedroom]."

   e.g. 2 – "I will [read] every weeknight at [8:45pm] in [my bed].

Main message:

"Take care of your body. It's the only place you have to live."
– Jim Rohn

WEEK 21 – Healthy Habits – Nutrition

PERMAH ELEMENT

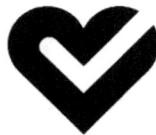

Health

Rationale

We are what we eat, and we need food as fuel for our bodies. Everything we eat has a short and long-term health effect on our bodies. The food choices we make affect our health, mood, energy and physical appearance. Food is the source of energy for all parts of our bodies and directly affects how our body and mind work.

A balanced diet consists of plant foods, such as vegetables and fruit, grain-based foods as well as moderate amounts of animal foods, such as lean meat and dairy products. Before we eat something, it helps to ask ourselves the question: Is this food going to give my body good energy or empty energy?

Drinking water is also extremely important for our bodies – not having enough fluid in our body can cause headaches, fatigue, make us feel cranky and affect our concentration. Water helps keep our body temperature stable, it carries nutrients and oxygen to our cells, cushions joints, protects organs and tissues and removes waste.

When we make healthy food and hydration choices, we are more likely to enjoy wellness in our body and mind, we will have more energy for being active, we will have better sleep as a result and the cycle will continue.

Teachers to read and facilitate the following with the class:

Description of Personal Wellbeing Practice: Nutrition

1. Think of one easy healthy food option you could have as a snack when you are hungry (after school or on the weekend when you are at home).
2. Now finish this sentence for what you are going to eat at a time you are usually hungry. "I will eat [INSERT FOOD CHOICE] when I am hungry each day at [TIME] in [PLACE]."
   e.g. I will eat [a banana] when I am hungry at [4:00pm] in [the kitchen].
3. Think of a time when you could have an extra drink of water or have water instead of another drink.
4. Now finish this sentence "I will have an extra drink of water each day at [TIME] in [PLACE]."
   e.g. "I will have an extra drink of water [every morning when I get up] in [the kitchen]."

Main message:

"Every time we eat is an opportunity to nourish our bodies."
– Author Unknown

WEEK 22 – Password Goals

PERMAH ELEMENT

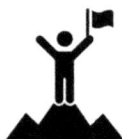

Accomplishment

Equipment required (optional)

Laptop, tablet, mobile phone or computer to use to set passwords.

Rationale

To get the most out of this next semester we should revisit and change our password goals. Regardless of where we are with our goals for the year, we can all benefit from hitting pause midway through the year and taking a closer look at where we are and where we are wanting to go.

We should note what has gone well and what needs more attention. We should reflect and be proud of what we have achieved so far – big or small. It all takes work and we should consider the impact of our efforts so far.

Research in the fields of neuroscience and psychology shows that goal setting actually works. If we don't take the time to figure out what we want in our lives, we just float along. A useful way to fast track our goals is to create a goal orientated password to unlock our devices. We unlock our devices several times each day, therefore it is a way to be frequently reminded of our goals – particularly when we are in autopilot mode typing our passwords.

Setting a password goal reminds us of what we are striving for, bringing our top priority goal into focus, every time we unlock our devices. This seemingly small act, repeated over and over, can go a long way toward helping us stay on task with achieving our goals. By changing our passwords to reinforce a goal we are trying to accomplish, we will put it top of mind and unconsciously focus in on ways to make those things happen (Adams-Miller 2017). We should re-evaluate our goals, make adjustments and remember our 'why' for the goals we are setting.

Teachers to read and facilitate the following with the class:

Description of Personal Wellbeing Practice: New password goals

1. Think of two things you were really happy with last semester and one thing you would like to improve on this semester.
2. Share this with your elbow partner (the person beside one of your elbows)!
3. Next, reflect on your last password goal (for those who did this with UPP's PWP in term 1). Were you able to achieve your goal? What could you do differently this time? Share with the person next to you.
4. Decide what your top priority goal is for this semester (it could be to do with school work; relationships, extracurricular, etc).
5. Next, make your goal password-ready (but do not share this password). Be creative. Use shorthand, abbreviations, numbers. For example, if you want to achieve certain grades (3Bs and 2Cs in Semester 2), it could be 3B2Csem2; or if you want to make the district cricket team, your

password goal could be districts2020. Other examples are: try1newthing2day 20pushups 1actofkindness.

6. If you have access to a device, take the time now to change your password. Otherwise, do this later today.

Main message:

"Your goals are the roadmaps that guide you and show you what is possible for your life." – Les Brown

WEEK 23 – Introduction to Meaning

PERMAH ELEMENT

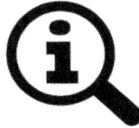

Meaning

Rationale

As humans, we desire meaning and purpose in our lives. We want a reason for what we do and we want it to matter. A meaningful life consists of belonging to and serving something that we believe is bigger than ourselves (Seligman 2011). When we have a sense of meaning and purpose, we are happier, more motivated, more committed and more satisfied.

To find meaning we need to work out what our highest strengths are and use our strengths in the service of something we believe is larger than we are. We usually draw meaning from multiple sources, including family and love, work, religion and various personal projects (Emmons 1997).

To find meaning we need to look for the positive difference we are making for others in our daily lives. How we think about the task we are doing is more important than the task itself. For example, a cleaner at the hospital could feel that they are just sweeping floors and emptying bins; another might think they are working a job that will pay their bills and feed their family, another might think they are building a career that will lead to other opportunities and yet another might feel that they are fulfilling a calling that helps people to recover from illnesses by ridding the hospital of germs.

Teachers to read and facilitate the following with the class:

Description of Personal Wellbeing Practice:
Make the mundane meaningful (McQuaid & Kern 2017).

1. Think of a task that you find meaningless. It might be doing your chores, it might be a subject at school or time spent doing something you didn't choose.
2. Now ask yourself "What could be the purpose of this task?" "What would happen if I didn't do this task at all? (Or if no one ever did this task?)" and "How could this task possibly help me in the future, or how could it help someone or something else?"
3. Write down all your answers so you can see the bigger value of a little task.

Main message:

"It's not what you do, but how much love you put into it that matters."
– Rick Warren

WEEK 24 – Live your Legacy

PERMAH ELEMENT

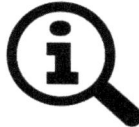

Meaning

Rationale

Research has uncovered that meaning can be found through many paths which include having a sense of belonging, having a purpose that motivates us to serve others, having a story to help us make sense of our place in the world and having experiences that lift us above the everyday and connect us to something bigger (Smith 2017).

Meaning and purpose usually surface over time; however, spending time thinking about what you want your meaning in life to be can help guide you in the right direction. We also need to step back from the daily details and look at the bigger picture in a positive way – this can ignite a sense of hope and pull us into action (McQuaid & Kern 2017).

Teachers to read and facilitate the following with the class:

Description of Personal Wellbeing Practice: Live your Legacy

1. As a class, brainstorm some positive values, personal characteristics and contributions to humanity that would make / have made a positive difference in the world.

2. Imagine that one day after you have passed, one of your grandchildren asks about you and your life.

3. Write a brief summary of how you would personally like to be remembered and described, using some values, personal characteristics and contributions to humanity that really stand out for you.

4. Your challenge for this week is to try to live with that sense of meaning and purpose straight away. Start living your legacy now.

Main message:

"Act as though what you do makes a difference. It does."
– William James

WEEK 25 – Awe-Inspiring

PERMAH ELEMENT

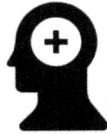

Positive Emotion   *Relationships*

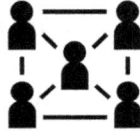

Rationale

When we experience something that is awe-inspiring for us, we can feel connected to something bigger than ourselves. These times of transcendence are rare moments that lift us above the hustle and bustle of our daily lives. In these moments, our sense of self fades away, along with our worries and desires and we can feel deeply connected to other people and things in the world (Smith 2017).

We can be inspired by a beautiful sunrise, by art or music, witnessing an act of kindness or being in a state of flow doing what we love. These transcendent experiences can change us. One study had students look up at a tall eucalyptus tree for one minute; afterwards they felt less self-centered, and they even behaved more generously when given the chance to help someone (Smith 2017). Studies show spending time in nature can provide perspective, reminding us that we are part of a much bigger world (Zhang, Piff & Iyer 2014). Life can make more sense when we have moments of transcendence and we experience a state of peace and wellbeing.

Teachers to read and facilitate the following with the class:

Description of Personal Wellbeing Practice: Awe-inspiring

1. Think of a time that you have experienced an awe-inspiring moment – a time when you witnessed beauty in the world. It could be in nature, in a museum, an act of moral courage or kindness, music, art or a person's story that inspired you.
2. Turn to the person next to you and share this experience with them and listen to their experience. Discuss what you were inspired by and how it made you feel.

Main message:

"People who have meaning in life are more resilient, they do better in school and at work, and they even live longer."
– Emily Esfahani Smith

WEEK 26 – Laugh out Loud

PERMAH ELEMENT

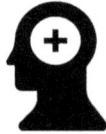

Positive Emotion   *Relationships*

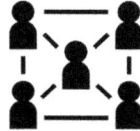

Rationale

Humour is a way we can boost our positive emotions. This can help us think better and be more creative. For example, a study showed doctors experiencing positive emotions made more accurate diagnoses (Seligman 2002). When we use humour we can see the lighter, brighter side to life and sustain a cheerful mood. Laughing has many benefits. Firstly, it is contagious – thanks to our mirror neurons, which make us respond to actions we observe in others. Laughing hard is a burst of exercise, triggering the release of endorphins that make us more relaxed both physically and emotionally.

Using humour to acknowledge mistakes without becoming angry or frustrated plays an important role in developing our resilience. While humour can be fun and help us feel better, it must never be used to hurt someone. We should laugh *with* people not *at* people. Humour increases levels of social support through reducing conflict and enhancing positive feelings towards others (Martin 2001).

The benefits of laughing occur whether the laugh is real or fake – the body cannot tell the difference. By seeking opportunities for humour and laughter we can improve our emotional health, strengthen our relationships and find greater wellbeing.

Teachers to read and facilitate the following with the class:

Description of Personal Wellbeing Practice:
Laugh out Loud (LOL)

1. Students are to gather in a circle.
2. We are going to hear a joke and the challenge for everyone is to respond with wild laughing – real or fake – as the body doesn't know the difference. The fake laughing usually leads to real laughing anyway.
3. Teacher to ask for someone to lead the group in a joke (explain joke suitability for this group – nothing rude or degrading) or there are some options below.
   - Why can you never trust an atom? Because they make up everything.
   - What did the left eye say to the right eye? Between us, something smells.
   - How do you make a tissue dance? Put a little boogie into it.
   - I asked my daughter if she'd seen my newspaper. She told me that newspapers are old school. She said that people use tablets nowadays and handed me her iPad. The fly didn't stand a chance.
   - Why was 6 afraid of 7? Because 7,8,9.
4. Consider sharing: At first this might have been awkward or tricky. But after some time, the jokes (possibly even the bad ones) and laughter may have led to some positive emotion, relationships and wellbeing for members of the group.

Main message:

"A good laugh overcomes more difficulties and dissipates more dark clouds than any other one thing." – Laura Ingalls Wilder

WEEK 27 – Gratitude Letter

PERMAH ELEMENT

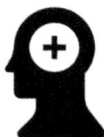

Positive Emotion   **Relationships**

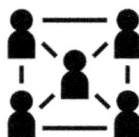

Rationale

Research has shown that grateful people experience higher levels of positive emotions such as joy, enthusiasm, love, happiness and optimism. The practice of gratitude as a discipline can protect us from feeling jealous, greedy, resentful or bitter (Emmons 2007).

In being grateful, we recognise the goodness in our life and we acknowledge that the source of much goodness is from outside ourselves. We can be grateful for someone, something or a situation. It can be felt as a sense of wonder in noticing and appreciating the ordinary things in life. When we take things for granted our gratefulness is inhibited.

Gratitude is not just an attitude; it is also a choice. It is choosing gratitude that enables us to receive. Gratitude can motivate us to repay the goodness we have been given (Emmons 2007). When we acknowledge that others have supported and helped us in big or small ways, we benefit from the positive emotions and wellbeing that being grateful gives us.

Teachers to read and facilitate the following with the class:

Description of Personal Wellbeing Practice: Gratitude Letter

1. Think of a person whom you would like to meaningfully thank. This person may have helped you, been kind to you or had a positive influence in your life (and they may continue to do so). It might be a friend, teacher, family member, coach or relative.
2. Write a short letter to this person expressing your appreciation for how they have impacted you. Include in detail what you are thanking them for and why it helped you.
3. Once you have finished the letter (which you might need to do at home), deliver the letter to the person, or call them and read the letter to them.

(If it is not possible to give the letter or call the person – the process of writing the letter itself is enough to increase your wellbeing.)

Main message:

"The single greatest thing you can do to change your life today would be to start being grateful for what you have right now."
– Oprah Winfrey

WEEK 28 – Sharing our Grateful Moments

PERMAH ELEMENT

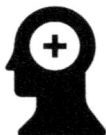

Positive Emotion

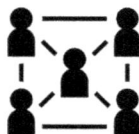

Relationships

Rationale

It is well documented that there are many benefits to practising gratitude. The expression of gratitude is associated with happiness, wellbeing, life satisfaction, optimism, forgiveness, enthusiasm and love (Emmons 2007). Sharing and acknowledging what we are grateful for is one of the most powerful of all positive psychology tools. Research has found it to increase happiness and decrease depressive symptoms for up to six months (Seligman et al 2005).

Teachers to read and facilitate the following with the class:

Description of Personal Wellbeing Practice:
Sharing our grateful moments with others

1. Think about a moment in your life that you are grateful for. It can be big or small.
2. Share this moment with your elbow partner. Explain how it made you feel and why it happened.
3. Practise active listening (see ACR in PWP WEEK 13) while your partner shares. Ask them one follow-up question about their moment, and invite them to share a little more.

Main message:

"Happiness is the only thing that multiplies when you share it."
— Albert Schweitzer

WEEK 29 – Three-minute Stress Buster

PERMAH ELEMENT

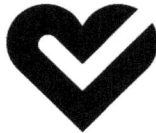

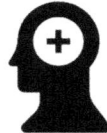

Health   *Positive Emotion*

Equipment required
- Some space for students to move on the spot
- A clock, watch or phone for timing

Rationale

Stress is a state of mental, physical or emotional tension, resulting from demanding circumstances. At different times in our lives (especially near the end of term), we all experience demanding circumstances resulting in stress – but it is not always a bad thing. It can sharpen our focus, as well as increase stamina and alertness to help us rise to the challenges we face.

There are two different types of stress – one is good or productive stress and the other is negative or distress. Good stress (eustress) is when we feel uncomfortable, nervous and pressured but believe we can handle it. It can be energising, improve our performance and usually only lasts a short time (Lazarus 1966). It can also inspire us to take action (finish the assignment, sort out the friendship issue).

We might have this stress before an exam or an athletic race, when meeting new people or when trying something new. If we notice that we are feeling stressed, we can realise that our bodies are telling us that something is important to us, and we can respond to the motivation and energy it provides. When we are able to cope with difficult and challenging situations, new learning, growth and connection will often come out as a result (McQuaid & Kern 2017).

We can't avoid all stress in our lives. Instead, we are better off finding ways to cope with the stressors that are bound to come our way as we journey through life. Some useful strategies for coping with stress are: mindfulness, visualisation, being organised, journaling, drawing, deep breathing, listening to relaxing music, dancing and exercise. We'll try a few that might help this week.

NB: There may be times when we feel negative stress is overwhelming, and at these times we should seek the support and guidance of family, trusted adult friends, school teachers or counsellors, or youth health organisations like Beyond Blue, ReachOut or Headspace.

Teachers to read and facilitate the following with the class:

Description of Personal Wellbeing Practice:
3-minute Stress Buster
1-minute exercise, 1-minute mindfulness and 1-minute deep breathing.

1. First, we are going to get our heart rates up by **moving our bodies for 1 minute**.
2. Start by running on the spot for 15 seconds. Next, jump up and down on the spot and shake your arms and whole body for 15 seconds. Star jumps for 15 seconds. Freestyle dance for 15 seconds.
3. Then stop and **count your pulse for 1 minute as a mindful activity**. (Younger students may just observe the way the body feels after the exercise.) Notice the way your body feels,

notice how strong your pulse is and how it starts to slow down again as time goes on.

4. Now sit or lie down where you are and close your eyes. We are going to use **deep breathing to calm our minds and bodies for one minute**. Place your hands on your belly and slowly breathe in through your nose. Breathe deeply so the breath moves your hands slightly. Then slowly breathe out, contracting your abdominal muscles to gently push the air out.

5. Breathe in to the count of four and breathe out for the count of four. Continue for 1 minute.

Once you have tried this three-minute stress buster, consider which of the three activities was the most helpful to you (and you might like to use it over the next couple of weeks). As we are all unique, different stress relieving strategies will work better for us than others. We need to try different strategies to find what works best for us (Lyubomirsky 2014). This is called 'person-activity fit.'

Main message:

"You can't control the wind, but you can adjust the sails."
– Thomas S Monson

WEEK 30 – Mindful Walking

PERMAH ELEMENT

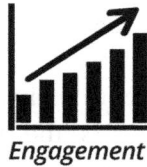

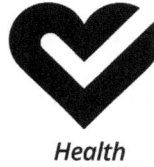

Engagement   *Health*

Equipment required

A large space inside or outside for students to walk around without coming into contact with each other or objects. It could be a verandah, eating area, oval or laps of the classroom.

Rationale

Mindfulness, at its simplest, is the training of attention. With enough training, our attention can become calm and focused (Tan 2012). Through mindfulness our minds can become clear and calm, and our natural state of happiness emerges.

There is an analogy we can use – think of our mind as a snow globe that is being shaken – the 'snow' particles (our thoughts) are floating everywhere. When we stop shaking the globe, the white 'snow' particles settle and the fluid inside becomes clear.

Each day, our minds can be in a constant state of snowing with thoughts and feelings. When we train ourselves in mindfulness, we can learn to let the snow particles fall and settle. Then we can have more clarity in our mind.

Mindfulness is present moment awareness. It is observing what is going on in and around us, without judging anything or getting carried away by the pressures that we experience (Snel 2013). Mindfulness can be in the form of feeling the sun on our skin, noticing the smell of the air or feeling a ripple of frustration in our body. We are to pay attention to our experiences, but not hold on to them or create a negative story about them.

Being mindful involves effort and intentionality. Research shows that mindfulness can lead to reduced stress and anxiety, improved sleep, greater self-awareness, less anger and frustration, increased confidence, better relationships, improved capacity for focus and concentration, better learning and greater levels of enjoyment in life (Greco et al 2005; Semple et al 2006).

Teacher to read and facilitate the following with the class:

Description of Personal Wellbeing Practice: Mindful Walking

To practise mindful walking, we are going to make a line standing one behind the other and with at least an arm's length between each person. There should be a designated leader at the front so everyone can follow the same path. Either do laps of the room/area or continue in a straight line. The practice should be three – five minutes long.

1. We start by standing still. Become aware of your body and how it feels. Notice your posture, feel the weight of your body pressing down toward the ground, and your heels pushing into your shoes. Be aware of all the subtle movements that are keeping you balanced and upright.
2. Now begin to walk more slowly than normal pace. With each step, be aware of the gentle heel-to-toe rhythm as each foot makes contact with the ground. Carefully notice your

foot, inside your sock, inside your shoe. Walk softly as if you are walking on eggshells.

3. Be aware of each movement that is made, feeling the thigh muscle lift the leg and move it into the next position, feeling the foot coming off the floor and setting it back down, feeling your arms and hands in the air. Focus on the right side for a few steps and then focus on the left side for a few steps.

4. When your thoughts begin to wander away from your movement, note the thought, and use your mindfulness 'muscles' to return your focus back to your experience of your body walking. It is the coming back and returning to your practice that is the training of attention.

5. It is now time to allow yourself to come to a gentle stop. Once again experiencing yourself standing still – as you feel the earth beneath your feet.

Main message:

"Training your mind to be in the present moment is the #1 key to making healthier choices." – Susan Albers

WEEK 31 – Savouring the Moment

PERMAH ELEMENT

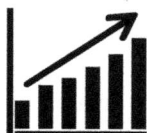

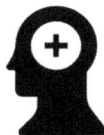

Engagement   **Positive Emotion**

Rationale

If you savour an experience, it is like swishing the experience around ... in your mind (Bryant & Veroff 2006). When we slow down to notice and appreciate the good things we are experiencing, we can increase our happiness and our wellbeing (Seligman 2002). To savour something, we need to pay attention and enjoy what we are experiencing. We allow ourselves to get totally immersed in it, using all of our senses. Savouring intensifies and extends the positive experience. If we eat something delicious and don't savour it, we sometimes miss out on the enjoyment of it.

We can savour things in the present moment, things that have happened in the past, or things we are looking forward to in the future. Being able to tune in and use our senses to savour things allows us to fully experience and enjoy the good things that life has to offer. By deliberately prolonging the positive experiences in our lives with savouring (through reliving, enjoying the moment and looking forward to the future), we can enjoy the benefits of greater happiness and boosted wellbeing in the short and long-term (Bryant & Veroff 2006).

Teachers to read and facilitate the following with the class:

Description of Personal Wellbeing Practice:
Savouring the Moment

1. Find something to savour right now in the present moment. Use your senses to find something that you are experiencing now that is enjoyable. It might be the sound of a bird outside, an object in the room that you are interested in, the feeling of your hands resting in your lap, the sunshine or breeze coming in through a window or just relaxing and sitting quietly. Nothing else is required of you right now except to notice something and appreciate it.

2. Your challenge is to notice something (which can be large or small) and transform it into something even better by becoming fully immersed in it. Notice, pay attention and appreciate what you are experiencing right now. We will be silent for one minute and savour.

3. For further savouring delights, commit to savouring one other experience today. It can be an enjoyable meal, a run or walk in nature, washing your hands, listening to your favourite music or a conversation with one of your favourite people. All you need to do is slow down, notice, appreciate and enjoy.

Main message:

"Ultimately, time is all you have, and the idea isn't to save it, but to savour it." – Ellen Goodman

WEEK 32 – Broaden and Build Brainstorm

PERMAH ELEMENT

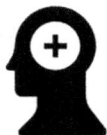

Positive Emotion   *Relationships*

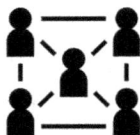

Rationale

The 'broaden and build' theory states that positive emotions broaden our awareness and encourage creative, original and exploratory thoughts and actions (Fredrickson 2004). When we are experiencing positive feelings, we can think more quickly and creatively. Our mind broadens due to enhanced neural connections. This is caused by the release of dopamine and serotonin, which are neurochemicals that make us feel good. Positivity also broadens our social responses – allowing us to connect and relate better to others. Over time, this builds our resources and capacity for wellbeing.

On the other hand, when we are experiencing negative emotions, the mind constricts and focuses in on the imposing threat (real or imagined). This limits our ability to be open to new ideas and build resources and relationships (Fredrickson 2009). Positive emotions expand our awareness and allow us to take in more of our surroundings and contextual information than we can during neutral or negative states (Garland et al 2015). We need both ways of responding at different times. In threatening situations, we need to be quick acting and narrowly focused.

However, if the threat is not real or lasting it can be detrimental to our health to stay in this responsive state. The broaden and build theory helps us to understand that we can use positive emotions to be more creative and calm in our problem solving, in our friendships (especially when things are tense), in our schoolwork and other interests. Little moments of positivity, although fleeting, can reshape who we are by setting us on a path of growth and building our enduring resources for a healthy life (Garland et al 2015).

Teachers to read and facilitate the following with the class:

Description of Personal Wellbeing Practice:
Broaden and Build Brainstorm

Divide the class into five teams (4-6 students per team)

1. Individually, think of something that makes you feel happy. It might be a place, a person, a great memory, a beautiful picture, your favourite music or meal. Spend a few moments with those happy thoughts. (You don't need to share these with anyone.) The goal here is simply to increase positive emotion so that we are able to broaden and build more effectively in a group activity.
2. Next, we are going to brainstorm as a group. Each team will be judged on quantity of responses, as well as creativity, teamwork, humour and the appropriateness of the responses.
3. All groups are given three minutes to brainstorm and come up with appropriate solutions to the question: **What would be the possible consequences if there was no night? (i.e. if night time did not exist ... ever.)**
4. When I say 'go', the aim is to generate as many responses as you can as a group and nominate a group scribe to record them. There is no right or wrong response here. "Go."

5. Each team can share their responses with the class in order to determine which team was most effective in this challenge.

6. Class discussion – how may boosting positive emotions (as per Step 1 of this PWP) have helped us with our creativity and awareness in this activity?

Main message:

"Just as water lilies retract when sunlight fades, so do our minds when positivity fades." – Barbara Fredrickson

WEEK 33 – Overcoming Negativity Bias

PERMAH ELEMENT

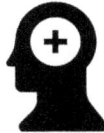

Positive Emotion

Rationale

Negativity bias is the human tendency to notice and be more influenced by bad things and bad experiences, instead of neutral or positive experiences. Examples of our negativity bias include remembering a bad day more easily than a good day, or remembering insults instead of the nice things people say. Our brains react more strongly to negative input than positive input.

We have a negativity bias because humans evolved to notice and respond more forcibly to the bad – this actually helped our ancestors stay alive. Negative emotions focus our energy for survival, which is fine if there is a lion in the classroom. While it is unlikely that a lion would be in the classroom, our brains are still wired to be constantly on the lookout for harm or danger. In most cases, this is unhelpful in our modern-day world.

Left unchecked, the negativity bias can get in the way of our happiness and wellbeing.

Knowing that we have a negativity bias can help us balance our negativity with positivity. We need much more positivity to outweigh the negativity in order to flourish.

Because our brains are like Velcro for negative experiences, and like Teflon (the stuff that makes frying pans non-stick) for positive ones, we need to intentionally notice and savour the positive experiences and feelings we have (Hanson 2010). We need three, four, five or six positive emotions to outweigh one negative emotion. The exact ratio is hard to determine (Brown, Sokal & Friedman 2013) and will be different for everyone.

Within bounds, higher positivity ratios are predictive of flourishing mental health (Fredrickson 2013). Steps to increase positives include: scattering your day with things that you will enjoy, keeping a gratitude journal and savouring the good.

Teachers to read and facilitate the following with the class:

Description of Personal Wellbeing Practice: Overcoming Negativity Bias

Using the Losada Positivity Ratio (that tells us that each negative interaction needs to be 'balanced' by at least three positive interactions) can be a great guide in practically overcoming our negativity bias. It can help us put things into perspective and not be swayed by our sensitivity to negatives.

1. On your paper draw a line down the middle.
2. Think about your day yesterday.
3. Reflect on one negative experience that happened and write it down on one side of the line.
4. Now think of some positive experiences and choose three to write down on the other side of the paper.

5. Spend a moment savouring the positive emotions from the good things that happened yesterday.

Using a ratio can help us balance out our tendency to notice the bad, and we can intentionally look for more positives. This is also really important in our relationships. We can increase the positivity in our relationships by using the ratio as a guide and always trying to outweigh the one negative with three to six positives.

Main message:

"By taking just a few extra seconds to stay with a positive experience, you'll help turn a passing mental state into a lasting one."
– Adapted from a quote by Rick Hanson

WEEK 34 – Best Possible Self and Dream Job

PERMAH ELEMENT

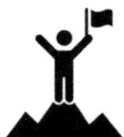

Accomplishment   **Positive Emotion**

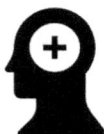

Rationale

The focus of attention on both the good and the possible can produce a burst of inspiration (Boniwell 2012). Thinking and writing optimistically about our future can increase our positive emotions and enhance wellbeing in a sustainable way (Sheldon & Lyubomirsky 2006). This is because optimism is born out of a positive expectation of our future. Developing an optimistic viewpoint has many advantages, including being more healthy, having less stress, being more adaptive and being able to apply continuous effort. If we think that the future can be positive, we are more willing to put in time and energy to make that come about (Segerstrom 2014).

Teachers to read and facilitate the following with the class:

Description of Personal Wellbeing Practice: Best Possible Self and Dream Job

1. We are going to spend three minutes visualising our best possible self and dream job and then we will write down what we imagined.
2. Sitting quietly, close your eyes.

3. Spend three minutes thinking about yourself in 10 years' time. Think that everything has gone as well as it possibly could; that you have achieved what you aimed for; that you are the best possible version of yourself. Visualise yourself working in your dream job and what that looks like. Imagine you have worked hard and have all of what you had hoped for. You are where you wanted to be at this stage. You are the sort of person that you want to be. Think about what you have studied or what skills you have gained, where you are living and how you are feeling about your life.

4. Now spend a few minutes writing down what you envisioned for your best possible self and job.

Main message:

"Optimism is the faith that leads to achievement; nothing can be done without hope and confidence." – Helen Keller

WEEK 35 – Happy Memory Building

PERMAH ELEMENT

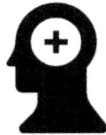

Positive Emotion   *Relationships*

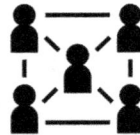

Rationale

Memories are powerful. Our memories actively shape our experiences, our relationships and what we want for our future. We know that we are more likely to remember negative experiences than positives ones due to our negativity bias. This can be helpful, as by remembering the things that caused us trouble in the past, we are more likely to avoid them in future. Research has found we can create more positive emotions in our lives by reliving and strengthening our wonderful, happy memories (Catalino & Fredrickson 2011).

With deliberate effort we can use our good memories to increase our wellbeing. While reliving the positive memory may feel short and fleeting, it is like putting money in the bank. Positive emotions accrue and help build your emotional, intellectual, social and physical resources. Positive emotions enable a broadened mindset, which seems to be the basis for the discovery of new knowledge, new relationships and new skills – all of which lead to more positive emotions (McQuaid & Kern 2017).

When we remember and savour our positive memories, we increase our positive emotions. These include feelings of gratitude, serenity, fulfilment, joy, wonder, amusement and love. These positive emotions change the way our minds and our bodies work. They change the very nature of who we are, down to our cells (Fredrickson 2011) – transforming our outlook on life and our ability to face challenges. The science of positive emotions is key to helping people deal with adversity and live a meaningful life (Fredrickson 2011).

Teachers to read and facilitate the following with the class:

Description of Personal Wellbeing Practice:
Happy Memory Building

1. Think of a great, feel-good memory that you shared with another person.
2. Relive that memory in your mind. Think about where you were, what you could see, what you could hear, or any smells or tastes you remember.
3. Think about what the other person was doing and try to remember their face and how they looked and what you thought they may have been feeling.
4. Think about the best part of the whole memory.
5. Remember how you felt and spend a few moments feeling all the positive emotions you experienced in that moment.
6. Next time you see the person, share the memory with them. Explain how much you value the memory – tell them what you remember about it so they can enjoy reliving it with you. If this feels awkward, use this sentence starter: "Hey, the other day I was thinking about …"

If it is not possible to talk in person, call or email them. If that person is no longer with us, share this memory with someone else who knew and cared for them.

Main message:

"Positive emotions don't just make us feel good, they transform our minds, our bodies and our ability to bounce back from hard times."
– Barbara Fredrickson

WEEK 36 – Your Superhero Strengths

PERMAH ELEMENT

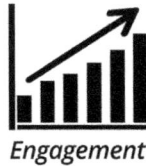

Engagement

Rationale

We all have positive character traits to be discovered, valued, used and further developed. Working in our strengths is energising. Character strengths are about how you relate to other people and the world around you. They are different from talents, skills or knowledge; strengths are valued for moral and intrinsic reasons, whereas talents are valued for their tangible outcomes (Peterson & Seligman 2004).

Our character is made up of lots of different strengths and everyone has a different set of strengths including things like curiosity, bravery, kindness, humour and hope. (See a full list of VIA [Values in Action] character strengths below.) Knowing our strengths and using them every day can lead to increased performance, as well as feeling more confident and satisfied with life. They are the things we are good at and enjoy doing (McQuaid & Lawn 2014). Using and developing our strengths allows us to work with the way our brain is already wired to perform at its best (Buckingham & Clifton 2001).

To become aware of our strengths, we are able to reflect on our best moments and identify what strengths we were drawing on in those times. Using a strengths test can help as well. (A free 10-minute youth strengths test for ages 10 -17 is available from the Trustees of Pennsylvania University, at https://strengthsprofile.com/en-gb/. Note that students will need to register individually if they would like to do this test.) Studies have shown that it is important to develop and celebrate our strengths, as it can prevent negative outcomes while increasing positive development and thriving (Peterson & Park 2009).

Teachers to read and facilitate the following with the class:

Description of Personal Wellbeing Practice:
Your Superhero Strengths

1. Think of a time when you have been proud of yourself. Alternatively, imagine a future situation that would make you feel proud.
2. Reflect on what personal character strengths you may have used to get to that point (e.g. to win a prize you may have needed a love of learning and perseverance in training/studying; to stand up for someone else, you may have used kindness and bravery; to change your idea about someone you may have used open-mindedness, appreciation and fairness.)
3. Teachers may assist by reading out the list of Character Strengths below during the above step.
4. Now focus on only two or three character strengths that you may have used in that situation.
5. Allow yourself to have a bit of fun with this activity. We are going to draw a superhero with those two or three particular strengths as superpowers. Think about how those strengths could serve as a force for good in our world.

6. Name your superhero and its superpowers. You might also like to give your superhero a prop- like Wonder Woman's lasso of truth. Some other ideas to get you thinking are: gratitude = flower; fairness = scales; love of learning = book; curiosity = magnifying glass.

Alphabetised list of VIA (Values in Action) Character Strengths

Appreciation	Gratitude	Open-mindedness
Bravery	Honesty	Perseverance
Caution	Hope/Optimism	Perspective
Creativity	Humour	Self Control
Curiosity	Kindness	Sociability
Enthusiasm	Leadership	Spirituality
Fairness	Love	Teamwork
Forgiveness	Love of learning	

Main message:

"What lies behind us and what lies before us are tiny matters, compared to what lies within us." – Ralph Waldo Emerson

WEEK 37 – Mindfulness Strategies

PERMAH ELEMENT

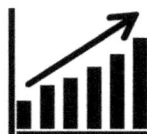

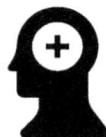

Engagement   *Positive Emotion*

Rationale

Mindfulness is "to pay attention, on purpose, to the present moment" (Grossman 2015). The positive benefits of mindfulness have been proven across a number of studies. Being mindful can reduce stress and anxiety, increase concentration and engagement, lead to better sleep, improve social skills and help develop problem-solving and decision-making skills (Jones, Greenberg & Crowley 2015). Mindfulness is an active practice that requires us to focus our mind's eye in that moment. We can do this by giving our full attention to what we are doing at that moment.

The reason mindfulness is so effective is that it goes beyond our conceptual mind and helps calm our nervous system – which is subject to overstimulation and negative stress. Regular mindfulness training gives us an opportunity to respond to, instead of react to, our environment. "Under duress we don't rise to our expectations, we fall to our level of training." Bruce Lee.

Teachers to read and facilitate the following with the class:

Description of Personal Wellbeing Practice: Mindful Strategies

For mindfulness activities we use the five Ss. Sitting straight, Still, Silently, Soft breathing and Shut eyes.

Star Hand Trace

1. Spread the fingers out on one hand like a star.
2. Use the index finger on your other hand to trace the outline of your star hand.
3. Take a deep breath in as you move to the top of your thumb.
4. Breathe out as you move down between your thumb and first finger.
5. Take another breath in as you move to the top of your first finger.
6. Breathe out as you move down between your first and second fingers.
7. Repeat until you have taken five slow, deep breaths.
8. When finished, go back to the start and repeat the whole process.

Senses Countdown – Open your eyes, but remain seated in your place...

Think of:
- 5 things you can see;
- 4 things you can touch;
- 3 things you can hear;
- 2 things you can smell;
- 1 thing you can taste.

Main message:

"Peace. It does not mean to be in a place where there is no noise, trouble or hard work. It means to be in the midst of those things and still be calm in your heart." – Unknown

WEEK 38 – Kindness Catching

PERMAH ELEMENT

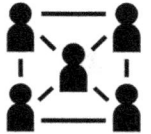

Relationships   *Positive Emotion*

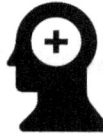

Rationale

Kindness can be defined as the quality of being friendly, generous and considerate. Affection, gentleness, warmth, concern and care are all associated with kindness. People who are kind and compassionate are usually the most successful (Brooks 2011). Kindness is an interpersonal skill and can be learned through trained repetition. Being kind to others improves our wellbeing and connectedness and makes us happier (Lyubomirsky 2008).

There are many ways to bring about the benefits of kindness into our lives. We can perform random acts of kindness, or write down when people show kindness to us. We can also perform acts of kindness that are not random, but are deliberately directed towards others, when we notice an opportunity.

Another very powerful way for us to foster more kindness in our lives is to think of times that we ourselves have been kind to others. In a study done by Adam Grant at Wharton Business school (2013), people who were asked to remember the times that they themselves had been kind gave more generously to others than those people who were asked to remember times when others had been kind to them. Recalling our actions of kindness helps us reinforce and build a vivid self-image of ourselves as a kind person. We then find ways to live up to the 'kind person' image and become more kind.

Teachers to read and facilitate the following with the class:

Description of Personal Wellbeing Practice: Kindness Catching

1. Think of three times that you have been kind to others in the past.
2. Go through each of the three memories and visualise them in your mind. Think of the way you felt at the time and how the person responded to your kindness. ·
3. Now write down those three times when you have been kind, giving as many details as you remember.
4. Share one of these with your shoulder partner.

Main message:

"Those who bring sunshine to the lives of others cannot keep it from themselves." – James M Barrie

WEEK 39 – Forgiveness with Loving-Kindness Meditation

PERMAH ELEMENT

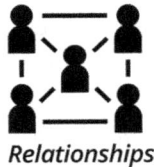

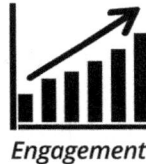

Relationships   *Engagement*

Rationale

Forgiveness can be defined as a shift in thinking. It means we don't wish harm to the person who hurt us; instead we wish good things for them. There is not always reconciliation and it is not pardoning, condoning or excusing the behaviour (Lyubomirsky 2007). When we forgive, we don't need to forget, but we do need to choose not to let the other person's actions control our emotions or actions.

Forgiveness is an important part of good relationships. Forgiveness is hard and takes a great deal of courage. "Forgiveness is the attribute of the strong," according to Gandhi. If we don't forgive, we hold a grudge, which interferes with our ability to feel close to other people. Empirically validated studies document the positive effects of forgiveness including less anger, more optimism and better health (Seligman 2002).

We can learn to be more empathetic and develop compassion by forgiving others. A good place to start might be with small things. To help us forgive, we can wish good things or no harm to the person. This will help us understand that we can choose to work on our feelings towards others (Eades 2008).

One way to build our forgiveness and compassion 'muscles' is the Loving-Kindness meditation. This focuses on developing feelings of goodwill, kindness and warmth towards others (Salzberg 1997). Loving-kindness meditation has been found to increase love, joy, contentment, gratitude, pride, hope, interest, amusement, awe (Fredrickson et al 2008) and positive emotions (Kok et al 2013).

Teachers to read and facilitate the following with the class:

Description of Personal Wellbeing Practice: Loving-Kindness Meditation

In the loving-kindness meditation, we are going to offer ourselves and those around us love and kindness. We are going to repeat, after the meditation leader, four mantras silently to ourselves.

1. Find a place to sit either in a chair or on the floor.
2. We will use the five Ss for our meditation practice. Sitting straight, Still, Silently, Soft breathing and Shut eyes.
3. Take some slow, deep breaths through your nose, into your belly. Feel your body start to soften as you trigger your relaxation response.
4. Bring your attention to your nose. As you inhale, feel the cool air going in, and as you exhale, feel the warm air going out.
5. See yourself in a kind, gentle way. Imagine you are talking to yourself. By opening your heart to yourself you will begin to see the positive energy you create within and around yourself. When your heart is full and you are peaceful, you will be able to send those same feelings into the world. Repeat each line after me (silently, in your own mind):

May I be well,
May I be happy,
May I be peaceful, (if it is helpful – think of how much joy and happiness you could cause yourself and others, with a peaceful mind),
May I let go of anger and sadness.

6. Now think of a good friend. Imagine their face and repeat each line after me:
   May they be well,
   May they be happy,
   May they be peaceful,
   May they let go of anger and sadness.

7. Now think about someone in school or a sibling that you sometimes find challenging and repeat each line (in your mind):
   May they be well,
   May they be happy,
   May they be peaceful,
   May they let go of anger and sadness.

8. Now think of all living things and repeat each line:
   May they be well,
   May they be happy,
   May they be peaceful,
   May they let go of anger and sadness.

9. Finally bring your love and kindness back to yourself and repeat each line after me:
   May I be well,
   May I be happy,
   May I be peaceful,
   May I let go of anger and sadness.

10. Bring your awareness back to your breathing. Take three slow breaths, then open your eyes.

Main message:

"Love creates a communion with life. Love expands us, connects us, sweetens us, ennobles us." – Jack Kornfield

WEEK 40 – Shout-outs – Relationships matter

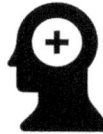

PERMAH ELEMENT

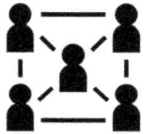

Relationships **Positive Emotion**

Rationale

Having a sense of belonging and feeling connected socially are vital for wellbeing. It leads to higher self-esteem, greater life satisfaction, lower levels of stress, less mental illness and longer life (Smith 2017). Good relationships take time and energy to develop and maintain, but they are well worth the effort. When we genuinely show others respect and appreciation, we are meeting a basic need and helping them flourish (Fredrickson 2013).

Today (as we near the end of the year), we have a wonderful opportunity to let someone know that we have noticed them do something we respect or appreciate. This will not only benefit the person you offer a shout-out to, but increase your wellbeing, too.

Teachers to read and facilitate the following with the class:

Description of Personal Wellbeing Practice: Shout-outs

1. Think of a time this year that someone in the room has done something that you respected or appreciated. It can be big

or small. Think about what they did, why you admired that action and how it made you feel.

2. Write it down.

3. We are now going to give you the opportunity to share your 'shout-out' with the group. Be sure to look at the person and use their name.

Main message:

"Appreciation is a wonderful thing. It makes what is excellent in others belong to us as well." – Voltaire

2.2 Primary Schools Personal Wellbeing Practices

The following are PWPs that have been written specifically with primary school students in mind. You may like to focus on one of the PERMAH elements each term. Or instead, you may prefer to try a broad range of activities each term. Teachers who are wanting to provide a debrief or explanation to the students are encouraged to read the relevant section of this book in Part 1. Below, we have simply focussed on the ways to make it practical.

Positive emotions

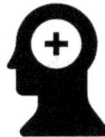

Positive Emotion

- **Kindness.** Do something that is kind for someone today. It might be saying something kind, including them in your game, offering to take their rubbish to the bin.
- **Gratitude.** Think of something that you are grateful for. It can be very simple like a tree you noticed or the breakfast you ate this morning or a smile your friend gave you. Teacher to choose for students to either write it down, draw it or share with a partner.

- **Happiness.** Think of something that makes you laugh or smile. It might be a funny book, joke, movie or a time with a friend or family member that made you happy. Teacher to choose for students to either write it down, draw it or share with a partner.

Engagement

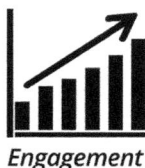

Engagement

- **Flow activities.** Rub your tummy and pat your head. Air performances: students give imaginary performances at teacher's instructions – for example, air guitar, air skipping, air juggling, air tennis, air piano.
- **Mindfulness activities.** We use the 5 Ss. Sitting straight, Still, Silently, Soft breathing and Shut eyes.
  - Building on this, we have included two mindfulness activities from which to choose.

Star Hand Trace

1. Spread one hand out like a star.
2. Use the index finger on your other hand to trace the outline of your star hand.
3. Take a deep breath in as you move to the top of your thumb.
4. Breathe out as you move down between your thumb and first finger.
5. Take another breath in as you move to the top of your first finger.
6. Breathe out as you move down between your first and second fingers.

7. Repeat until you have taken five slow, deep breaths.
8. When finished, go back to the start and repeat the whole process.

Senses Countdown – open your eyes, but remain seated in your place...
Think of:
   a) 5 things you can see;
   b) 4 things you can touch;
   c) 3 things you can hear;
   d) 2 things you can smell;
   e) 1 thing you can taste.

Relationships

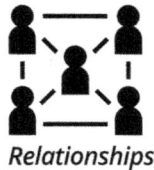

Relationships

- **Kindness catching.** Think of a time that someone has been kind to you and think of a time that you have been kind to someone else. Write them down or draw a picture.
- **Shout-out.** Think of someone in your class who has done something that you admire or respect. Teacher to choose whether students stand up and give the shout-out or write it down or draw a picture and then give it to that person. Tell them what they did and why you admire or respect them for the action they took. Be sure to look at the person and use their name.
- **Listening.** Share a memory with a partner of your favourite holiday or time with your family. Listen carefully by giving your partner your eye contact and attention. Seek more information from your partner by asking a question.

Meaning

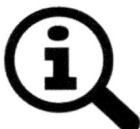

Meaning

- **Be awed by nature.** Go outside and choose a natural object and look at it. It could be a tree, insect, cloud, flower or blade of grass. Notice its colour, texture, shape and movement. Reflect on how everything belongs and is part of this world.
- **Purpose.** Imagine you had the power to change the world. You could change it by cleaning up the environment, helping the poor or finding a cure for diseases. Think about how you would want to change the world; what would you do? Teacher to choose for students to either write it down, draw it or share with a partner.
- **Belonging.** Think of a way in which you contribute and belong to the school community. It might be participating in sports days, supporting your team, being involved in music or a club. It might be the way you help other classmates or take pride in the school grounds. Now think of something extra you could do to help the school community. Teacher to choose for students to either write it down, draw it or share with a partner.

Accomplishment

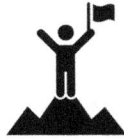

Accomplishment

- **Grit.** What is the hardest thing you have done in the last month? Teacher to choose for students to either write it down, draw it or share with a partner. Acknowledge that we can do hard things when they come our way.
- **Confidence.** Strike a power pose. Pretend that you are Wonder Woman or Superman. Stand tall with your hands on your hips and head up high. Stay in this position for one minute, feeling strong and confident.
- **Practice makes progress.** Choose one thing that you want to practise more to make progress. Teacher to choose for students to either write it down, draw it or share with a partner.
- **Neuroplasticity.** Our brain can learn and grow. Practise catching a tennis ball with your non-preferred hand for a few minutes or write your name with your less dominant hand any time you do it this week. Notice how challenging it is to do something that we have not had much practice doing. If you keep at it, notice the improvement over time as your brain adapts to the practice.

Health

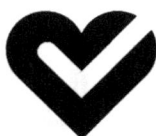

Health

- **Increase heart rate.** Start by running on the spot for 15 seconds. Next, jump up and down on the spot and shake your arms and whole body for 15 seconds. Star jumps for 15 seconds. Freestyle dance for 15 seconds.
- **Calm body.** Sit or lie down where you are and close your eyes. We are going to use deep breathing to calm our minds and bodies for one minute. Place your hands on your tummy and breathe slowly in through your nose. Breathe deeply so the breath moves your hands slightly. Then slowly breathe out, contracting your tummy muscles to gently push the air out. Breathe in to the count of four and breathe out for the count of four. Continue for 1 minute.

2.3 Whole School Wellbeing Events And Ideas

The following list includes some simple ideas for actions that can be taken by a whole school community (in order to engage both staff and students). Some of them are one-off events, while others are ongoing in nature. Not all ideas will be relevant or helpful in your school context, but are included in order to get your 'creative juices flowing'. The list is not comprehensive – it is simply more a brainstorm. One helpful use for this list of ideas is to take to a Wellbeing or PERMAH committee meeting in order to stimulate conversation about what is the best fit for your own school context.

1. Create a **Wellbeing Poster week** – give students time during one lesson at school this week to design their own poster that reflects one aspect of Wellbeing and Positive Education that they have found to be helpful.
2. **Quote sharing** – Find a quote that is related to one aspect of Wellbeing and Positive Education and share it with your class, explaining why it resonates with you.
3. **TED talks** can be held in the school hall by teachers or students who wish to contribute on a topic within Wellbeing and Positive Education.
4. Watch the Disney Pixar movie **'Inside Out'** (in the school hall during lunchtime for a week) and discuss the value of the different emotions, back in class.
5. **Grow your mind day** – choose one day each semester (or year) where students have an extended lunch and are encouraged to give something a go that they have never tried

before. Invite staff or students with particular interests to set up activities for students and staff to have a go. It's great when staff attempt the activities and model what you want to see from students.

6. Name the **school fish** or **school bird** in order to build community and connection – in guidance counsellor or Principal's office, etc.

7. **Mindful Monday or Chilled Out Tuesday etc** – start off each week by setting up a space with a number of mindful activities for staff or students to access at their leisure during one of the break times (or before/after school). Activities could include mandalas, guided meditation CD, mindful eating (bring your food and sit in quiet), gratitude (five finger gratitude, or journaling), BYO reading. It would be a silent space with different options in the room for people to enjoy, be mindful, find some space in their lives and centre themselves.

2.4 Staff Personal Wellbeing Practices

The following ideas might be useful to issue as challenges to your staff, as you journey with Wellbeing and Positive Education. I would encourage schools not to attempt too much. Start small, win and build momentum. Don't commit to doing things for a whole term. Maybe just try one fortnight or one week with a focus on one of these things. Allow it to be driven by a team or a group of early adopters, rather than just the same single person each time.

Consideration should also be given to challenges set outside of work hours – obviously they won't be taken up as readily as those that we can commit some time to (think meeting time). If we want to send a message to our teachers that we really value their wellbeing, maybe we could commit 10 minutes once a month (or term) to one of the practices below. This is the educator's equivalent of putting our money where our mouth is. We've got to 'walk the talk'.

We achieve more together than we do on our own, so make sure you're not the only one banging the drum. The other key here is don't commit to banging the drum for long periods of time. As we all know, there are times of the term when people may be less open to trying something in this realm. It is also worth considering making some of these things optional, so that people can participate at the level that they feel capable (also recognising what we know about 'person-activity' fit – explained in Section 1). Some people might detest your best ideas and love others. If our goal is to encourage people to engage, it would be wise to consider some optional activities and others that are mandated (however, I suggest that as much as possible, work time or meeting time is given for those requirements).

The other key here is that I don't believe that more is better. The perfectionists reading this book must beware. Do not try to do them all. It will just cause you to be overwhelmed. It would be more helpful to take on one challenge that you feel ready for, and then do that one as well as you can. If it helps, keep doing it. If it doesn't, try something else. We are all different. The list below shows simple tools. Just choose one and go for it.

Positive emotion

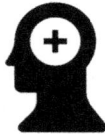

Positive Emotion

- Set up a **gratitude wall/board** in the staff room for 'three good things today' and encourage staff to write up their three things each day (only do for a short period, before people lose interest and it goes stale).
- Choose one week each term and make it a **'gratitude email week'.** Each staff member is encouraged to express their gratitude towards one other person in an email. Aim to recognise someone who has done something noteworthy or excellent.

Engagement

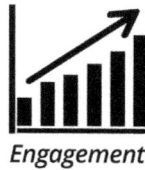

Engagement

Name your strengths – during a staff meeting, use the Gallup Strengths Finder (Rath 2001) or the free VIA Survey (2019) to identify your current strengths. Then each staff member can make a plan to use one of their main strengths in the next week.

Relationships

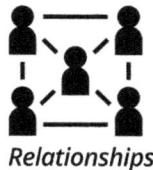

Relationships

- Have a **shared lunch** once a month with your department/ whole staff where everyone brings a plate (or the school provides afternoon tea).
- **Authentic compliment week** – Watch the clip: 'NAB Credit Cards Commercial – Honesty' (NAB 2012) at the end of a staff meeting. Discuss how they "Shone a light on what is right." Give someone an HSAC this week – honest, specific, authentic, compliment.
- **Mystery staff member** – staff are allocated another staff member for a semester. They are asked to look for good things their nominated person does and write them an anonymous letter at the end of the semester describing the two things

they noticed them do and the impact that had on other people. Don't reveal who your person is.

- **Secret friend** – Building on the previous idea, at the beginning of the year staff are asked if they would like to participate in Secret Friend – an initiative led by a Senior School teacher. Volunteers then provide their birth date, favourite colour, favourite flower and five things that make them smile. This information is then sent to their secret friend. Throughout the year, staff leave anonymous messages, gifts and surprises for their secret friend. These can bring joy, warmth and a real sense of belonging throughout a busy school year.

- **Team building** – We recently took our team to Laser Zone and the stories they tell bring a great deal of positive emotion and strengthen relationships. Well worth the investment and energy.

- **Meetup Groups** – Lunchtime and after school meetups can take place for a variety of activities. One group might meet to make crafts, another for book club, stand-up paddle boarding, bike riding, meditation group, training together for a 10k run or Tough Mudder. N.B. Sharing interests and creating opportunities for staff to spend time together away from the regular work-focused conversation enables friendships to form and staff to feel a connection with their colleagues. Allow these groups to form and dissolve naturally based on interests and be aware how interest may ebb and flow. Don't push for attendance, just allow and encourage the opportunity for connection. They should be bottom-up initiatives, rather than top-down.

Meaning

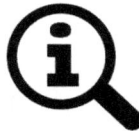

Meaning

- **Hands for the Community Day** – all staff spend a day volunteering at a local charity or not-for-profit organisation. Small work teams are formed to allow people to volunteer their time, energy and expertise for a backyard blitz for elderly residents of the community, or providing support to The Salvos, St Vinnies, Rotary Club or a local Aged Care Complex. In addition to the contribution that it makes in the community, staff can pursue their own sense of meaning and build relationships.

Accomplishment

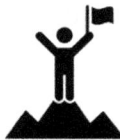

Accomplishment

- At the start of a year or term during a staff meeting, **watch 'Substitute Teacher – Mr Garvey – Key and Peele'** (Comedy Central 2016). **Share your story** with a colleague about a time you have found it difficult to understand or get to know your class. What did you do? What did you learn? What can you learn from each other?

- **My favourite mistake** – think about or write down the mistakes you have made in your work or life in the last couple of months that you have learned from. These are not your favourite mistakes because you made them, they are your favourites because you have learned from them. Record the lessons learned or insight gained.
- Get staff to link their **Personal Wellbeing plan** to their professional learning goal.

Health

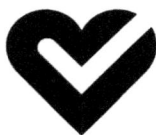

Health

- **Staff PD Expo** – two hours with staff on a PD day whereby staff choose from different workshops that enhance their wellbeing (e.g. lawn bowls, mandalas, gratitude walk, pizza making, board games, quiet reading, social tennis, yoga/mindfulness, baking in cooking rooms, calligraphy class).
- Use **fitballs as optional chairs** for staff in staffroom and lunch room. Bring some fun and physical activity into the everyday.

N.B. This list is not exhaustive. If you have some other ideas that have been successful in your school context, please send them through to us (admin@unleashingpersonalpotential.com.au), and we will continue to add to this inventory. This will make it even more helpful for schools in the future.

2.5 Wellbeing Education – The School Journey

The following is intended as a guide for the work that we do with schools in this space. It is intended as a guide only, and schools are encouraged to consult UPP in order to tailor the best implementation plan for your school journey of wellbeing and positive education. However, the following can give you a plan that you can use on your own, or with the support of UPP.

Exceptional incursions and workshops for students (targetted approach)

For exceptional incursions and workshops with your students (as short as 45 minutes, up to multiple days), please contact UPP and we can build an implementation plan with you. This approach works best for one whole cohort at a time (up to 250 students). We work with cohorts of students from year 5 to year 12 and cover various topics including wellbeing, PERMAH, leadership, growth mindsets, grit and positive peer relationships.

All UPP incursions use a learning, action, reflection process in order to ensure high engagement and interaction. The messages are relevant and practical strategies are always offered. All sessions also include online follow-up material.

These sessions are designed to help you launch Wellbeing with PERMAH in your school context in a way that engages, inspires and opens the minds of your students. These workshops / incursions tend to increase buy-in of the students (and also the teachers who will support them with the follow-up lessons) for the journey ahead.

Following these incursions / workshops, facilitated by UPP, the online PWP's or lessons are then an incredibly helpful tool, to ensure the students revisit and deepen their learnings, and continue to build on their toolbook of wellbeing practices.

Reach out to us if you'd like to look at some options and create a plan of attack for your school.

Whole school approach

Some schools prefer a whole school approach- including engaging staff and students in a sequential way. The below process is an overview of a typical process that schools can follow. You will note that we use the model of learn it, live it, teach it and embed it (Hoare, Bott & Robinson, 2017).

LEARN IT AND LIVE IT (YEAR 1)

1. **Survey staff** using PERMAH Workplace survey (http://www.unleashingpersonalpotential.com.au/permah-survey) and collate all data.
2. We will then immediately send each person a personalised **Personal Wellbeing report,** which gives them a measure of their wellbeing in each of the 6 PERMAH elements.
3. UPP two to three hour Workshop- **An Introduction to Wellbeing with PERMAH** with all staff.
4. Included in workshop - Review of personalised teacher Personal Wellbeing report. Each person creates a **Personal Wellbeing plan**. People are able to select from the range of

strategies that may help to boost the PERMAH Element they would most like to improve, based on our toolkit of PWPs and other interventions.

5. Relevant follow-up material (online access to all Personal Wellbeing Practices for all staff) provided after session.

6. **Post-Survey Teachers** – using the PERMAH workplace survey and collate all data regarding notable changes.

Notes:

- There is no charge for administering the Survey and providing the related reports.
- Books may be purchased, which will allow staff to learn about all areas at their own discretion.
- All UPP Personal Wellbeing Practices will be made available to all school staff during (and following) the **Introduction to Wellbeing with PERMAH** session and for the remainder of the year, through the UPP website.
- UPP team member can be available regularly in order to check in on the progress of the initiative and adjust the planning and next steps as needed.

TEACH IT (YEAR 2)

1. SURVEY students using EPOCH youth survey and collate all data.

2. UPP Team to deliver Intro to Wellbeing with PERMAH to every cohort in the school (Involves one or two sessions per cohort). This approach works best for one whole cohort at a time (up to 250 students).

3. Students to select one intervention that they would like to implement.

4. Teachers use PWPs across the school with all students for the course of a year.

5. School to utilise UPP lesson plans and any others that are developed by the school.
6. At the end of the year, SURVEY students using EPOCH youth survey and collate all data.

EMBED IT (YEAR 2)

1. Staff to reflect regularly throughout year regarding existing whole-school practices that can be adjusted.
2. Staff to reflect regularly throughout year regarding personal or professional practices that can be adjusted. Continuation of personal wellbeing plan.
3. Departments and extra-curricular areas of the school consider practices that can be adjusted/improved to embed Wellbeing and Positive Education learnings.

CONTINUE TO LEARN, LIVE, TEACH AND EMBED IT (YEAR 2 AND BEYOND)

2.6 The Personal Journey – Where Do I Begin?

If you are an individual beginning this journey, all of these tools can be very overwhelming. We don't want paralysis by analysis. We want to keep it simple. Try the following steps:

1. Personally, if you are looking for one simple place to start, take the **PERMAH Workplace Survey (allow 10 minutes)**, available free of charge on our website – http://www. unleashingpersonalpotential.com.au/permah-survey. This will allow you to access a measure of your wellbeing across the PERMAH dimensions.
2. We will then immediately send you a personalised **Personal Wellbeing report**, which gives you a measure of your wellbeing in each of the 6 PERMAH elements.
3. In your PERMAH Survey report, you will be given a link to your **PERMAH builder**. This will allow you to:
   a) Choose the PERMAH area you would most like to improve.
   b) Choose your action steps – select from the range of strategies that may help to boost the PERMAH Element you would most like to work on, based on our toolkit of PWPs and other interventions.
   c) Create your own **Personal Wellbeing plan** (keep it small and simple to begin with).
4. **Review your results** and see how you are progressing by completing the PERMAH Workplace Survey again in a few months.

Support And Resources

If you work in a school, we may be able to assist you with:
- Student workshops and incursions- 45 minutes up to multiple days (including sessions on wellbeing, PERMAH, leadership, growth mindsets, grit and positive peer relationships)
- Teacher Professional Development
- Online Personal Wellbeing Practices

In order to hear from schools who have experienced working with UPP in the past, please visit our website to read some of their testimonials.

If you would like some support with your implementation plan, please contact us at admin@unleashingpersonalpotential.com.au.

We'd love to help your community THRIVE.

Whether your aim is to implement these practices in your own life, for your staff or team, or for your whole school, we wish you all the best.

From all of the team at Unleashing Personal Potential

References

ABS. (2013). *Causes of Death Australia.* Australian Bureau of Statistics. Canberra.

Achor, S. (2010). *The Happiness Advantage.* New York: Random House.

ACT. (2008). Key Facts: Cognitive and Noncognitive skills http://www. act.org/content/dam/act/unsecured/documents/WK-Brief-KeyFacts-CognitiveandNoncognitiveSkills.pdf

Adams-Miller, C. (2017). *Getting Grit, The evidence based approach to cultivating passion, perseverance and purpose.* Sounds True. Canada.

AIHW. (2011). Young Australians: their health and wellbeing. Australian Institute of Health and Welfare Cat. no. (PHE 140). Canberra: AIHW, p 593-602.

Ainsworth, M., Blehar, M., Waters E., & Wall, S. (1978). *Patterns of attachment: A psychological study of the strange situation.* Mahwah, NJ: Lawrence Erlbaum Associates, Inc.

Alarcon, G.M., Bowling, N.A. & Khazon, S. (2013). Great expectations: A meta-analytic examination of optimism and hope. Personality and Individual Differences. 54 (7): 821.

Algoe, S.B., Haidt, J., & Gable, S.L. (2008). Beyond reciprocity: Gratitude and relationships in everyday life. *Emotion.* 8(3), 425-429.

Al-Mabuk, R. & Enright, R. (1995). Forgiveness education with parentally love-deprived late adolescents. *Journal of Moral Education*. 24, 427–444.

American Psychological Association (2014.) Ten Ways to Build Resilience https://www.apa.org/helpcenter/road-resilience.aspx

Amabile, T.M. & Kramer, S.T. (2011). The Power of Small Wins. *Harvard Business Review* May.

Anderson, James (2018). Personal comment.

Ankin, L.B., Dunn, E. W., Norton, M.I. (2012). Happiness runs in a circular motion: Evidence for a positive feedback loop between prosocial spending and happiness. *Journal of Happiness Studies*. 13(2), 347-355.

Ankin, L.B., Dunn, E.W. & Norton, M.I. (2012). Happiness Runs in a Circular Motion: Evidence for a Positive Feedback Loop between Prosocial Spending and Happiness. *Journal of Happiness Studies*.

Ansel, K. (2009). Is your diet making you gain? Retrieved from www.health.msn.com.

Baer, R.A. (n.d.) Mindfulness Training as a Clinical Intervention: A Conceptual and Empirical Review. http://www.wisebrain.org/papers/MindfulnessPsyTx.pdf

Bandura, Albert (1982). Self-efficacy mechanism in human agency. *American Psychologist*. 37 (2): 122–147.

Barclay, E. (2014). Why Sugar Makes Us Feel So Good. Eating and Health https://www.npr.org/sections/thesalt/2014/01/15/262741403/why-sugar-makes-us-feel-so-good

Battersby, A. & Phillips, L. (2016). In the End It All Makes Sense Meaning in Life at Either End of the Adult Lifespan. https://doi.org/10.1177/0091415016647731

Bauman, A.E. (2004). Updating the evidence that physical activity is good for health: an epidemiological review 2000-2003. *Journal of Science and Medicine in Sport.* 2004 Apr;7(1 Suppl):6-19.

Baumeister, R. & Tierney, J. (2012). *Willpower: Rediscovering the Greatest Human Strength.* London: Penguin Group.

Baumeister, R., Bratslavsky, E., Finkenauer, C., & Vohs, K. (2001). Bad is stronger than good. *Review of General Psychology.* 323-370.

Benson, H. (1997). The relaxation response: therapeutic effect. Dec 1997 5;278(5344):1694-5. *Science* Vol. 278, Issue 5344, pp. 1693-1697 DOI: 10.1126/science.278.5344.1693-c

Ben-Shahar, T. (2007). *Happier: learn the secrets to daily joy and lasting fulfillment.* New York: McGraw-Hill. ISBN 0071510966. OCLC 176182574.

Berlin, J., & Colditz, G. (1990). A meta-analysis of physical activity in the prevention of coronary heart disease. *American Journal of Epidemiology.* 132: 612-28.

Berndt, T.J. (1992). Friendship and Friends' Influence in Adolescence. Association for Psychological Science. https://doi.org/10.1111/1467-8721.ep11510326

Berry, J.W., & Worthington, E.L. (2001). Forgivingness, relationship quality, stress while imagining relationship events, and physical and mental health. *Journal of Counseling Psychology.* 48, 447–455.10.1037/0022-0167.48.4.447.

Bertin, M. (2016). Mindful healthy mind healthy life.
https://www.mindful.org/body-scan-kid

Better Humans (2017). The Japanese Concept 'Ikigai' is a Formula for
Happiness and Meaning. https://betterhumans.coach.me/the-japanese-
concept-ikigai-is-a-formula-for-happiness-and-meaning-8e497e5afa99

Beyond Blue (2014). Workplace final report. https://www.headsup.org.au/
docs/default-source/resources/beyondblue_workplaceroi_finalreport_
may-2014.pdf

Beyond Blue (2015). The National Depression Initiative. MediaCom
Melbourne youthbeyondblue Anxiety and Depression Ad Tracking Survey
Post Campaign Research p 7.

Beyond Blue (2017). Help someone you know https://www.
youthbeyondblue.com/help-someone-you-know/supporting-a-friend

Beyond Blue Fact Sheet (2018). What is mental health? https://www.
beyondblue.org.au/the-facts/what-is-mental-health)

Biblica (2018). *The Bible New International Version* (NIV) https://www.
biblestudytools.com/niv/

Biswas-Diener, R., Kashdan, T., & Minhas, G. (2010). A dynamic
approach to psychological strength development and intervention. *Journal
of Positive Psychology.* 106-118.

Black, D.S., Milam, J., & Sussman, S. (2009). Sitting-meditation
interventions among youth: A review of treatment efficacy. *Pediatrics,*
124(3), 532–541.

Bolier, L., Haverman, M., Westerhof, G. H., Riper, H., Smit, F. &
Bohlmeijer, E. (2013). Positive psychology interventions: a meta-analysis

of randomized controlled studies. BMC Public Health. 13 (119). doi:10.1186/1471-2458-13-119.

Boniwell, I. (2012). *Positive Psychology in a Nutshell, The Science of Happiness.* Open University Press, England.

Borgonovi, F. (2008). Doing well by doing good. The relationship between formal volunteering and self-reported health and happiness. *Social Science and Medicine.* Jun;66(11):2321-34. doi: 10.1016/j.socscimed.2008.01.011.

Breus, M.J. (2013). Better Sleep Found by Exercising on a Regular Basis. https://www.psychologytoday.com/au/blog/sleep-newzzz/201309/better-sleep-found-exercising-regular-basis-0

Brewer, J., Worhunsky, P., Gray, J., Tang, Y., Weber, J. & Kober, H. (2011). Meditation experience is associated with differences in default mode network activity and connectivity. *Proceedings of the National Academy of Sciences of the United States of America.* 20254–20259.

Bridgeland, J., Bruce, M. & Hariharan, A. (2013) *The Missing Piece: A National Survey on How Social and Emotional Learning Can Empower Children and Transform Schools*: Washington, DC: Civic Enterprises.

Bronk, K.C. (2014). *Purpose in Life: A Critical Component of Optimal Youth Development.* Dordrecht: Springer.

Brown, B. (2010). *The Gifts of Imperfection.* Hazelden.

Brooks, D. (2011). *The Social Animal.* Random House.

Brown, B. (2012). *Daring Greatly: How the Courage to Be Vulnerable Transforms the Way We Live, Love, Parent, and Lead.* New York: Gotham.

Brown, N.J., Sokal, A.D. & Friedman, H.L. (2013). The complex dynamics of wishful thinking: the critical positivity ratio. *American Psychologist.* 68 (9): 801–13. arXiv:1307.7006. doi:10.1037/a0032850. PMID 23855896.

Bryant, F. & Veroff, J. (2006). *Savouring: a new model of positive experiences.* Marwan, NJ. Lawrence Erlbaum.

Buckingham, M. & Clifton, D.O. (2001). *Now, Discover Your Strengths.* Gallup Press.

Burke, Christine A. (2010). Mindfulness-Based Approaches with Children and Adolescents: A Preliminary Review of Current Research in an Emergent Field. *Journal of Child and Family Studies* April 2010, Volume 19, Issue 2, pp 133–144|.

Byrne, A. & Byrne, D.G. (1993). The effect of exercise on depression, anxiety and other mood states: a review. *Journal of Psychosomatic Research.* 13(3): 160-170.

Carver, C.S. & Scheier, M.F. (2002). Optimism. In Snyder, C.R. & Lopez, S.J. (Eds) *Handbook of positive psychology.* (pp 231–243).

Catalino, L. I., & Fredrickson, B. L. (2011). A Tuesday in the life of a flourisher: The role of positive emotional reactivity in optimal mental health. *Emotion.* 11(4), 938–950.

Chapman, G. (1992). *The five love languages: How to express heartfelt commitment to your mate.* Chicago, IL: Northfield Publishing.

Cheng, F.K. (2016). Is meditation conducive to mental wellbeing for adolescents? An integrative review for mental health nursing. *International Journal of Africa Nursing Sciences.* 4: 7–19. doi:10.1016/j. ijans.2016.01.001.

Ciarrochi, J., Kashdan, T.B. & Harris, R. (2013). The foundations of flourishing. In Kashdan, TB & Ciarrochi, J (Eds) *Mindfulness, acceptance, and positive psychology: The seven foundations of wellbeing.* (pp. 1-29). Oakland, CA, New Harbinger.

Cleary, T.J. (2011.) Emergence of self-regulated micro-analysis: Historical overview, essential features and implications for research and practice. In Zimmerman, B.J. & Schunk, D.H. (eds) *Handbook of regulation of learning and performance.* (pp 329-345). New York. Routledge.

Cohen, S. & Wills, T.A. (1985). Stress, social support, and the buffering hypothesis. *Psychological Bulletin*, 98(2), 310-357 San Diego, CA, US: Academic Press.

Colditz, G., Cannuscio, C. & Grazier, A. (1997.) Physical activity and reduced risk of colon cancer. *Cancer Causes and Control.* 8: 649-667.

Comedy Central (2016) Key and Peele: Substitute Teacher http://www.comedycentral.com.au/key-and-peele/videos/substitute-teacher

Compton, W.C., & Hoffman, E. (2013). *Positive Psychology: The Science of Happiness and Flourishing.* 2nd ed. Belmont, CA: Wadsworth Cengage Learning.

Cotton Bronk, K., Hill, P.L., Lapsley, D.K., Talib, T.L. & Finch, H. (2009). Purpose, hope, and life satisfaction in three age groups. pp 500-510 https://doi.org/10.1080/17439760903271439

Covey, S. (1989). *7 Habits of Highly Effective People.* Simon & Schuster.

Creswell, J.D. (2017). Mindfulness Interventions. *Annual Review of Psychology.* 68: 491–516. doi:10.1146/annurev-psych-042716-051139. PMID 27687118.

Csikszentmihalyi, M. (1997). *Finding flow: the psychology of engagement in everyday life*. New York: Basic Books.

Csikszentmihalyi, M. (2013). *Flow: The Psychology of Happiness*. Random House.

Csikszentmihalyi, M., Abuhamdeh, S. & Nakamura, J. (2005). Flow, in Elliot, A., *Handbook of Competence and Motivation*. New York: The Guilford Press, pp. 598–698.

Damon, W., Menon, J. & Cotton Bronk, K. (2003). The development of Purpose during adolescence. *Applied Developmental Science*. 7(3) pp 119-128.

Dana Foundation, The (2018). https://www.dana.org/brainglossary

Danner, D., Snowdon, D., & Friesen, W. (2001). Positive Emotions in Early Life and Longevity: Findings from the Nun Study. *Journal of Personality and Social Psychology*. 804-813.

Davidson, D.L. (1993). Forgiveness and narcissism: Consistency in experience across real and hypothetical situations. *Dissertation Abstracts International*. 54 27–46. Google Scholar.

Davidson R.J., Kabat-Zinn J., Schumacher J., Rosenkranz M., Muller D., Santorelli S.F., Urbanowski F., Harrington A., Bonus K. & Sheridan J.F. (2003). Alterations in Brain and Immune Function Produced by Mindfulness Meditation. *Psychosomatic Medicine*. Jul-Aug;65(4):564-70.

Davidson, R., & Lutz, A. (2008). Buddha's Brain: Neuroplasticity and Meditation. *IEEE Signal Processing Magazine*.

de Terte, I., Stephens, C. (2014). Psychological Resilience of Workers in High-Risk Occupations. *Stress and Health*. 30 (5): 353–355. doi:10.1002/smi.2627. ISSN 1532-3005.

Deatherage, G. (1975). The clinical use of "mindfulness" meditation techniques in short-term psychotherapy" (PDF). Journal of Transpersonal Psychology. 7 (2): 133–43.

DeLisi, M. (2014). Low Self-Control Is a Brain-Based Disorder. In *The Nurture Versus Biosocial Debate in Criminology: On the Origins of Criminal Behavior and Criminality* (Chapter 10) Edited by: Kevin M. Beaver, J.C. Barnes & Brian B. Boutwell SAGE Publications Ltd.

Dervic K., Oquendo, M.A., Grunebaum, M.F., Ellis, S., Burke, A.K. & Mann, J.J. (2004). Religious affiliation and suicide attempt. *American Journal of Psychiatry.* 2004;161(12):2303-8.

DeWall, C.N., Baumeister, R.F., Stillman, T.F. & Gailliot, M.T. (2007). Violence restrained: Effects of self-regulation and its depletion on aggression. *Journal of Experimental Social Psychology.* 43 (1): 62–76. doi:10.1016/j.jesp.2005.12.005.

Diamond. A. (2013). Executive functions. *Annual Review of Psychology.* 64: 135–168. doi:10.1146/annurev-psych-113011-143750. PMC 4084861. PMID 23020641.

Diener, E. (2003). Personality, culture and subjective wellbeing: Emotional and Cognitive Evaluations of Life Ed Diener. *Annual Review of Psychology.* 54:403–25 doi: 10.1146/annurev. psych.54.101601.145056

Diener, E. (ed) (2009). Assessing Well-Being: The Collected Works of Ed Diener. *Social Indicators Research Series* 39, DOI 10.1007/978-90-481-2354-4 10, C Springer Science+Business Media B.V. 2009.

Diener, E., & Biswas-Diener, R. (2008). *Happiness: unlocking the mysteries of psychological wealth.* Malden, MA: Wiley-Blackwell.

Diener, E., & Seligman, M. (2002). Very happy people. *Psychological Science*, 81-84. https://doi.org/10.1111/1467-9280.00415

Diener, E., Nickerson, C., Lucas, R., & Sandvik, E. (2002). Dispositional Affect and Job Outcomes. *Social indicators research.* pp 229-259.

Dimidjian, S. & Linehan, M.M. (2003). Defining an Agenda for Future Research on the Clinical Application of Mindfulness Practice. *Clinical Psychology Science and Practice.* Volume 10, Issue 2, June 2003, Pages 166-171.

Duckworth, A.L. (2007). Grit: perseverance and passion for long-term goals. *Journal of Personality and Social Psychology.* pp 1087-1101.

Duckworth, A.L. & Quinn, P.D. (2009). Development and Validation of the Short Grit Scale (Grit–S) *Journal of Personal Assessment.* Mar;91(2):166-74. doi: 10.1080/00223890802634290.

Duckworth, A.L. (2016). *The Power of Passion and Perseverance.* Scribner.

Duckworth, A., Grant, H., Loew, B., Oettingen, G., & Gollwitzer, P. (2011). Self-regulation strategies improve self-discipline in adolescents: benefits of mental contrasting and implementation intentions. *Educational Psychology.* 17-26.

Duhigg, C. (2013). *The Power of Habit.* London: Random House Books.

Dunn, A.L., Trivedi, M.H., Kampert, J.B., Camillia, G., Chambliss, H.O., Madhukar, L. (2005). Exercise treatment for depression – Efficacy and dose response. *American Journal of Preventive Medicine.* 28(1):1-8.

Durlak, J., Weissberg, R., Dymnicki, A., Taylor, R., & Schellinger, K (2011). The impact of enhancing students social and emotional learning:

a meta-analysis of school based universal interventions. *Child Development.* 405-432.

Dweck, C. (2006). Mindset: *The new psychology of success.* New York: Ballantine Books.

Dweck, C. (2009). Theories of Intelligence. htttp://www.education.com/reference/article/ theories-of-intelligence/

Eades, J. (2008). *Celebrating Strengths: Building Strength-based Schools.* Warwick. Capp Press.

Eccles, J., Wigfield, A., and Schiefele, U. (2001). Motivation to succeed. In N. Eisenberg, *Handbook of Child Psychology* (pp. 1017-1095). New York: Wiley.

Eckert, T.L. & Hinze, J.L. (2000) Behavioral conceptions and applications of acceptability: Issues related to service delivery and research. *School Psychology Quarterly. 15(2).*

Edmunds, W.J. (1997). Social Ties and Susceptibility to the Common Cold. *The Journal of the American Medical Association.* 278 (15): 1231, author reply 1232. *doi:10.1001/jama.1997.03550150035018. PMID 9333253.*

Elias, M., Zins, J., Weissberg, R., Frey, K., Greenberg, M., Haynes, N., Kessler, R., Schwab-Stone, M., & Shriver, T. (1997). *Promoting social and emotional learning: guidelines for educators.* Alexandria, VA: Association for Supervision and Curriculum Development.

Elliot, A.J., Sheldon, K.M. & Church, M. (1997). Avoidance personal goals and subjective wellbeing. *Personality and Social Psychology Bulletin.* 23: 915-927.

Emmons, R. (n.d.). *Gratitude and wellbeing.* http://emmons.faculty. ucdavis.edu/gratitude -and-wellbeing/

Emmons, R.A. (1997). *Handbook of Personality Psychology* Academic Press. pp 485-512.

Emmons, R. (2007). *Thanks! How the new science of gratitude can make you happier.* New York: Houghton Mifflin.

Emmons, R.A. (2010). Why Gratitude is Good. *Greater Good Magazine.* Berkeley https://greatergood.berkeley.edu/article/item/why_gratitude_is_good

Emmons, R., & McCullough, M. (2003). Counting blessings versus burdens: An experimental investigation of gratitude and subjective wellbeing in daily life. *Journal of Personality and Social Psychology,* 377-389.

Fehr, E. & Gächter, S. (2000). Fairness and Retaliation: The Economics of Reciprocity. *Journal of Economic Perspectives* 14(3) pp 159-181.

Fells, A. (2016). Australians are spending more on mental health services and employers need to take notice http://theconversation.com/australians-are-spending-more-on-mental-health – services-and-employers-need-to-take-notice-53642

Flade, P., Asplund, J. & Elliot, G. (2015). Employees Who Use Their Strengths Outperform Those Who Don't. *Workplace* Oct 8, 2015.

Ford, C. (2018). Six Tips for Self Kindness Institute of Positive Education. Geelong Grammar School https://www.ggs.vic.edu.au/institute/blog/blog-posts/six-tips-for-self-kindness? j=12900andsfmc_sub=238092678andl=19_HTMLandu=262215andmid=100001875andjb=17

Fox K.C., Nijeboer S., Dixon M.L., Floman J.L., Ellamil M., Rumak S.P., Sedlmeier P. & Christoff K. (2014). Is meditation associated with altered brain structure? A systematic review and meta-analysis of morphometric neuroimaging in meditation practitioners. *Neuroscience and Biobehavioral Reviews*. 43: 48–73. *doi:10.1016/j.neubiorev.2014.03.016. PMID 24705269.*

Frankl, V. (1992). *Man's search for meaning: An introduction to logotherapy* (I. Lasch, Trans.) Boston: Beacon.

Fredrickson, B.L. (2001). The role of positive emotions in positive psychology – the broaden and build theory of positive emotions. *The American Psychologist* 56 (3), 218-226.

Fredrickson, B. L. (2013). Positive emotions broaden and build. *Advances in Experimental Social Psychology, 47(1)*, 53.

Fredrickson, B.L., Cohn, M.A., Coffey, K.A., Pek, J. & Finkel, S.M. (2008). Open hearts build lives: positive emotions, induced through loving-kindness meditation, build consequential personal resources. *Journal of Personal and Social Psychology.* Nov;95(5):1045-1062. doi: 10.1037/a0013262.

Fredrickson, B. (2004). The broaden-and-build theory of positive emotions. *Philosophical transactions of the Royal Society of London. Series B, Biological sciences, 359*(1449), 1367-78.

Fredrickson, B. (2009). *Positivity: Groundbreaking research reveals how to embrace the hidden strength of positive emotions, overcome negativity, and thrive.* New York, NY, US: Crown Publishers/Random House.

Fredrickson, B.L., & Losada, M.F. (2005). Positive affect and complex dynamics of human flourishing. *American Psychologist, 60*, 678-686.

Fredrickson, B., & Branigan, C. (2005). Positive emotions broaden the scope of attention and thought – action repertoires. *Cognition and Emotion*, 313-332.

Friedenreich, C.M., McGregor, S.E., Courneya, K.S., Angyalfi, S.J. & Elliott, F.G. (2004). Case-control study of lifetime total physical activity and prostate cancer risk. *American Journal of Epidemiology.*159(8):740-9.

Froh, J.J., Miller, D.N., & Snyder, S. (2007). Gratitude in children and adolescents: Development, assessment, and school-based intervention. *School Psychology Forum*, 2, 1-13.

Froh, J.J., Kashdan, T.B., Yurkewicz, C., Fan, J., Allen, J. & Glowacki, J. (2010). The benefits of passion and absorption in activities: Engaged living in adolescents and its role in psychological wellbeing. *The Journal of Positive Psychology*, 5: 4, 311 — 332.

Gable, S., Gonzaga, G., & Strachman, A. (2006). Will you be there when things go right? Supportive responses to positive event disclosures. *Journal of Personality and Social Psychology*, 904-917.

Gaffney, M. (2011). *Flourishing.* London: Penguin Books.

Garland, E., Farb, N., Goldin, P. & Fredrickson, B.L. (2015). The Mindfulness-to-Meaning Theory: Extensions, Applications, and Challenges at the Attention–Appraisal–Emotion Interface in Psychological Inquiry 26(4):377-387.

Gollwitzer, P.M. (1990). Action phases and mind-sets. In Higgins, E Tory; Sorrentino, Richard M. *Handbook of motivation and cognition: foundations of social behavior.* 2. New York: Guilford Press. pp. 53–92. ISBN 978-0898624328. OCLC 12837968.

Gollwitzer, P.M. (1999). Implementation intentions: strong effects of simple plans. *American Psychologist*, 493-503.

Good, C., Aronson, J., & Inzlicht, M. (2003). Improving adolescents' standardized test performance: An intervention to reduce the effects of stereotype threat. *Applied Developmental Psychology*, 645 – 662.

Gottman, J. (2002). *The relationship cure: strengthening your marriage, family and friendships.* Harmony Books.

Grammar, G. (n.d.). *What is positive education?* Retrieved from Geelong Grammar: https://www.ggs.vic.edu.au/School/Positive-Education/What-is-Positive-Education

Grant, A. (2013). *Give and Take.* Great Britain, Weidenfeld & Nicolson.

Greco, L.A., Blackledge, J.T., Coyne, L.W., & Enreheich, J. (2005). Integrating acceptance and mindfulness into treatments for child and adolescent anxiety disorders: Acceptance and Commitment Therapy as an example. In S. M. Orsillo & L. Roemer (Eds.), *Acceptance and Mindfulness-Based Approaches to Anxiety: Conceptualization and Treatment.* New York: Kluwer/Plenum.

Grossman, P. (2015) Mindfulness: Awareness formed by an embodied ethic. *Mindfulness* 6(1) 17-22

Gu, J., Strauss, C., Bond, R. & Cavanagh, K. (2015). How do mindfulness-based cognitive therapy and mindfulness-based stress reduction improve mental health and wellbeing? A systematic review and meta-analysis of mediation studies. *Clinical Psychology Review.* 37: 1–12. *doi:10.1016/j.cpr.2015.01.006. PMID 25689576.*

Hakkarainen, R., Partonen, T., Haukka, J., Virtamo, J, Albanes, D & Lonnqvist, J. (2004). Food and nutrient intake in relation to mental wellbeing. Nutrition Journal. 2004; 3: 14. Published online 2004 Sep 13. doi: 10.1186/1475-2891-3-14.

Hanson, R. (2010) *Buddha's Brain: The Practical Neuroscience of Happiness, Love, and Wisdom*. New Harbinger Publications.

Harlow, H. (1958) The nature of love. *The American Psychologist.* 13 673-685.

Hartup, W. W., & Abecassis, M. (2002). Friends and enemies. In P. K. Smith & C. H. Hart (Eds.), *Blackwell handbook of childhood social development* (pp. 286–306). Malden, MA: Blackwell.)

Harvard Medical School (2018). Understanding the stress response *Chronic activation of this survival mechanism impairs health* Harvard Health Publishing.

Hassed, C. (2008). *The Essence of Health: the seven pillars of wellbeing.* Sydney, Random House.

Hawker, D.S.J., & Boulton, M.J. (2000). Twenty years' research on peer victimization and psychosocial maladjustment: A meta-analytic review of cross-sectional studies. *Journal of Child Psychology and Psychiatry.* 41, 441-455.

Headspace. (2018). https://headspace.org.au/

Hebl, J.H., and Enright, R.D. (1993). Forgiveness as a psychotherapeutic goal with elderly females. *Psychotherapy: Theory, Research, Practice, Training, 30,* 658–667.10.1037/0033-3204.30.4.6

Hendren, R., Birrel Weisen, R. & Orley, J. 1994. *Mental Health Programmes in Schools.* Division of Mental Health, World Health Organisation: Geneva, Switzerland.

Hoare, E., Bott, D., and Robinson, J. (2017). Learn it, Live it, Teach it, Embed it: Implementing a whole school approach to foster positive mental health and wellbeing through Positive Education. *International Journal of Wellbeing*, 7(3), 56-71.

Hofmann, S., Grossman, P., & Hinton, D. (2011). Loving-kindness and compassion meditation: Potential for psychological interventions. *Clinical Psychology Review*, 1126-1132.

Hölzel B.K, Lazar, S.W, Gard, T., Schuman-Olivier, Z., Vago D.R. & Ott, U. (2011). How Does Mindfulness Meditation Work? Proposing Mechanisms of Action from a Conceptual and Neural Perspective. *Perspectives on Psychological Science.* 2011 Nov;6(6): pp 537-59 doi: 10.1177/1745691611419671.

Howell, A. (2009). Flourishing: achievement-related correlates of students' wellbeing. *Journal of Positive Psychology.* 1-13.

Hunter, J. P., & Csikszentmihalyi, M. (2003). The positive psychology of interested adolescents. *Journal of Youth and Adolescence.* 32, 27-35.

Huppert, F.A. & Johnson, D.M. (2010) A Controlled Trial of Mindfulness Training in Schools: The Importance of Practice for an Impact on Well-Being. *The Journal of Positive Psychology.* 5, 264-274. http://dx.doi.org/10.1080/17439761003794148

Huppert, F.A. & So, T.T.C. (2012). Flourishing across Europe: Application of a new conceptual framework for defining wellbeing. *Social Indicators Research.* 1-25.

Iacoboni, M. (2008). *Mirroring people.* New York: Picador.

Index, G.H. W. (2008). *Poll: Unhappy workers take more sick days.* Associated Press.

Institute of Positive Education, Geelong Grammar School, *Discovering Positive Education* manual.

Institute of Positive Education, Geelong Grammar School, *Discovering More Positive Education* manual.

James, W. (1890) Habit. *Principles of Psychology.* Vol 1. Ed. Frederick H. Burkhardt. Cambridge: Harvard UP, 1981. pp 109-31.

James, W. (1920). *Psychology: briefer course.* Harvard University Press.

Jones, D.E., Greenberg, M. & Crowley, M. (2015). Early Social-Emotional Functioning and Public Health: The Relationship Between Kindergarten Social Competence and Future Wellness *American Journal of Public Health* (Nov).

Jordan, J., Rand, D., Arbesman, S., Fowler, J., & Christakis, N. (2013). *Contagion of Cooperation in Static and Fluid Social Networks.* PLoS ONE.

Kabat-Zinn, J. (2003). Mindfulness based interventions in context: past present and future. Clinical Psychology: *Science and Practice.* 144-156.

Kabat-Zinn, J. (2013). *Full Catastrophe Living: Using the Wisdom of Your Body and Mind to Face Stress, Pain, and Illness.* New York: Bantam Dell.

Kahana, E., Tirth Bhatta, M.G.S., Lovegreen, L.D., Kahana, B., & Midlarsky, E. (2013). Altruism, Helping and Volunteering: Pathways to Well-Being in Late Life. *Journal of Aging and Health* Feb 25(1) 159-187.

Kahn, D. (2003). Montessori and Optimal Experience Research: toward building a comprehensive education reform. http://montessori-namta.org/PDF/kahnresearch.pdf

Kampert, J.B., Blair, S.N., Barlow, C.E. & Kohl, H.W. (1996) Physical activity, fitness and all cause and cancer mortality. *Annals of Epidemiology.* 6: 542-7.

Kaplan, D., Palitsky, R., Carey, A.L., Crane, T.E., Havens, C.M., Medrano, M.R., Reznik, S.J., Sbarra, D.A. & O'Connor, M.F. (2017). Maladaptive repetitive thought as a transdiagnostic phenomenon and treatment target: An integrative review. *Journal of Clinical Psychology.* 74 (7): 1126–36. doi:10.1002/jclp.22585. PMID 29342312.

Kasser, T. & Ryan, R. M. (1996). Further examining the American dream: Differential correlates of intrinsic and extrinsic goals. *Personality and Social Psychology Bulletin.* 22, 80–87.

Keng, S., Smoski, M.J. & Robins, C.J. (2011). Effects of mindfulness on psychological health: A review of empirical studies. *Clinical Psychology Review.* 31 (6): 1041–56. doi:10.1016/j.cpr.2011.04.006. PMC 3679190. PMID 21802619.

Kenhub (2018) Neurotransmitters https://www.kenhub.com/en/library/anatomy/neurotransmitters

Kern, M. (2016). *Professional Certificate in Positive Education – Subject 1 Introduction to Positive Education, Intensive 1 – Resources.* University of Melbourne.

Kessler, R.C., Berglund, P., Demler, O., Jin, R., Merikangas, K.R. & Walters, E.E. (2005). Lifetime prevalence and age-of-onset distributions of DSM-IV disorders in the National Comorbidity Survey Replication. *Archives of General Psychiatry.* 62: p. 593-602.

Keyes, Corey L.M. (2002). The Mental Health Continuum: From Languishing to Flourishing in Life. *Journal of Health and Social Behavior.* 43 (2): 207–222. doi:10.2307/3090197. ISSN 0022-1465.

Keyes, C.L. (2005) Mental illness and/or mental health? Investigating axioms of the complete state model of health. *Journal of Consulting and Clinical Psychology.* 73(3):539-48.

Koenig. H.G. Religion and medicine II: religion, mental health, and related behaviors. International Journal of Psychiatry in Medicine. 2001;31(1):97-109.

Kok, B.E., Coffey, K.A., Cohn, M.A., Catalino, L.I., Vacharkulksemsuk, T., Algoe, S.B., Brantley M & Fredrickson B.L. (2013). How positive emotions build physical health: perceived positive social connections account for the upward spiral between positive emotions and vagal tone. *Psychological Science.* July 2013 1;24(7) pp 1123-32. doi: 10.1177/0956797612470827.

Kotler, S. (2015). The Neurochemistry of Flow States, with Steven Kotler https://www.youtube. com/ watch?v=aHp2hkue8RQ

Kurth, F., Luders, E., Wu, B. & Black, D.S. (2014). Brain Gray Matter Changes Associated with Mindfulness Meditation in Older Adults: An Exploratory Pilot Study using Voxel-based Morphometry. *Neuro Open Journal.* 1 (1): 23–26. doi:10.17140/NOJ-1-106. PMC 4306280. PMID 25632405.

Lawrence, D., Johnson, S., Hafekost, J., Boterhoven De Haan, K., Sawyer, M., Ainley, J. & Zubrick S.R. (2015). *The Mental Health of Children and Adolescents. Report on the second Australian Child and Adolescent Survey of Mental Health and wellbeing.* Canberra: Department of Health.

Lazar, S., Kerr, C., Wasserman, R., Gray, J., Greve, D., Treadway, M. & Quinn, B. (2005). *Meditation experience is associated with increased cortical thickness.* Neuroreport, 1893-1897.

Lazarus, R.S. (1966). *Psychological Stress and the Coping Process.* New York, Toronto, London: McGraw-Hill Book Co.

Le Fevre, M., Kolt, G.S., Matheny, J. (2006). Eustress, distress and their interpretation in primary and secondary occupational stress management interventions: which way first? *Journal of Managerial Psychology.* 21 (6): 547–565. doi:10.1108/02683940610684391.

Libkuman, T.M., Otani, H., Kern, R.P., Viger, S.G. & Novak, N. (2007) Multidimensional normative ratings for the International Affective Picture System. *Behavior Research Methods, Instruments & Computers.* 39: 326-334.

Linley, A., & Harrington, S. (2004). Playing to your strengths. *The Psychologist.* https://thepsychologist.bps.org.uk/volume-19/edition-2/playing-your-strengths.

Locke, Edwin A.; Latham, Gary P (1990) *A theory of goal setting and task performance.* Englewood Cliffs, NJ: Prentice Hall. ISBN 978-0139131387. OCLC 20219875.

Lodish, H., Berk, A., Zipursky, S.L (2000). *Molecular Cell Biology: Section 21.4 Neurotransmitters, Synapses, and Impulse Transmission* (4th ed.) New York: W. H. Freeman.

Loehr, J. & Schwartz, T. (2005). *The Power of Full Engagement: Managing Energy, Not Time, Is the Key to High Performance and Personal Renewal.* Freeprint.

Losada, M., & Heaphy, E. (2004). The role of positivity and connectivity in the performance of business teams: A nonlinear dynamics model. *American Behavioral Scientist* 47(6), 740–765.

Lutz, A., Davidson, R.J. & Slagter, H.A. (2011). Mental Training as a Tool in the Neuroscientific Study of Brain and Cognitive Plasticity. *Frontiers in Human Neuroscience.* 5:17.

Lutz, A., Dunne, J. & Davidson, R. (2007). Meditation and the neuroscience of consciousness. In Zelazo, P., Moscovitch, M. & Thompson, E. *Cambridge Handbook of Consciousness.* Cambridge University Press.

Lyubomirsky, S., King, L., & Diener, E. (2005). The Benefits of Frequent Positive Affect: Does Happiness Lead to Success? *Psychological Bulletin,* 803-855.

Lyubomirsky, S. (2008). *The how of happiness: A scientific approach to getting the life you want.* New York: Penguin Press.

Lyubomirsky, S. (2014). *The Myths of Happiness: What Should Make You Happy, but Doesn't, What Shouldn't Make You Happy, but Does.* Penguin Books.

MacLeod, A.K., Coates, E. & Hetherton, J. (2008). Increasing wellbeing through teaching goal-setting and planning skills: results of a brief intervention. *Journal of Happiness Studies* Volume 9, Issue 2, pp 185–19.

Magyar-Moe, J.L. (2009) *Therapist's Guide to Positive Psychological Interventions.* Academic Press.

Mallough, R. (2013). An extra-large sized order of generosity. Retrieved from Macleans: http://www.macleans.ca/news/canada/an-extra-large-sized-order-of-generosity/

Maiorana, A., O'Driscoll, G., Cheetham, C., Collis, J., Goodman, C., Rankin, S., Taylor, R. & Green, D. (2000). Combined aerobic and resistance exercise training improves functional capacity and strength in chronic heart failure. *Journal of Applied Physiology.* 200;88:1565-70.

Martin, R. (2001). Humour, laughter and physical health. Methodological issues and research findings. *Psychological Bulletin.* 127: 504-19.

Maslow, A.H. (1970). *Motivation and Personality* (2nd ed.) New York: Harper & Row.

Mathers, C.D. & Loncar, D. (2006). Projections of global mortality and burden of disease from 2002 to 2030 *PLoS Medicine* 3 (11), e442.

Maxwell, K.A. (2002). Friends: The Role of Peer Influence Across Adolescent Risk Behaviors *Journal of Youth and Adolescence* Volume 31, Issue 4, pp 267–277.

McGonigal, K. (2012). *The willpower instinct: How self-control works, why it matters and what you can do to get more of it.* New York: Avery.

McKenna, L (2015). *Thrive: Unlocking the truth about student performance.* Brisbane.

McKnight, P.E. & Kashdan, T.B. (2009). – Purpose in life as a system that creates and sustains health and wellbeing: an integrative, testable theory. *Review of General Psychology,* 13 (3), 242-251.

McQuaid, M. & Kern, P. (2017). *Your Wellbeing Blueprint: Feeling good and doing well at work.* Michelle McQuaid Pty Ltd.

McQuaid, M.L. & Lawn, E. (2014). *Your Strengths Blueprint: How to be Engaged, Energized, and Happy at Work* https://www.amazon.com/Your-Strengths-Blueprint-Engaged-Energized /dp/0987271415 Michelle McQuaid Pty Ltd

Metts, S., & Cupach, W.R. (1998). Predictors of forgiveness following a relational transgression. Paper presented at the 9th International Conference on Personal Relationships, Saratoga Springs, NY.

Michie, D. (2008). *Hurry up and meditate.* Crows Nest: Allen & Unwin.

Mind matters (n.d.) – Module 1.3 p6 – https://www.mindmatters.edu. au/docs/default- source/learning – module-documents/mm_module1_3-protectiveriskfactors.pdf?sfvrsn=2

Muraven, M., Baumeister, R.F., & Tice, D.M. (1999.) Longitudinal Improvement of Self-Regulation Through Practice: Building Self-Control Strength Through Repeated Exercise. *Journal of Social Psychology.* 1999 Aug;139(4):446-57.

Murray, H.A. (1938). *Explorations in Personality.* New York: Oxford University Press p164.

Myers, D.G. (2000). The funds, friends, and faith of happy people. *American Psychologist*, 55, 56-67.

NAB (2012) Credit card commercial - honesty https://www.youtube.com/watch?v=CCWu1W9jNbk

Nakamura, J., & Csikszentmihalyi, M. (2014.) The concept of flow. In *Handbook of positive psychology.* 89-105. New York, NY: Oxford University Press.

Nakanishi, N. (1999) 'Ikigai' in older Japanese people. *Age and Ageing.* 28 (3): 323–324. doi:10.1093/ageing/28.3.323. ISSN 1468-2834.

Neal, D., Wood, W., & Quinn, J. (2006). Habits—A Repeat Performance. *Current Directions in Psychological Science.* https://dornsife.

usc.edu/assets/sites/545/docs/Wendy_Wood_ Research_ Articles/Habits/ Neal.Wood.Quinn.2006_Habits_a_repeat_performance.pdf198-202.

Neff K.D. & Dahm K.A. (2015). Self-Compassion: What It Is, What It Does, and How It Relates to Mindfulness. In: Ostafin B., Robinson M., Meier B (eds) *Handbook of Mindfulness and Self-Regulation*. Springer, New York, NY.

Neff, K.D. & McGehee, P. (2010); Self-compassion and Psychological Resilience Among Adolescents and Young Adults. *Self and Identity Journal*. Vol 9 2010 issue 3.

Neff, K. D., & Pommier, E. (2013). The relationship between self-compassion and other-focused concern among college undergraduates, community adults, and practicing meditators. *Self and Identity*. 12(2), 160-176.

Niemiec, R. (2017). Character Strengths Interventions: A Field Guide for Practitioners. Hogrefe Publishing.

Niemiec, R.M., Rashid, T., Linkins, M., Green, S., & Mayerson, N.H. (2013) Character strengths in practice. *IPPA Newsletter*. 5(4).

Norrish, J., Robinson, J. & Williams, P. (2011). *Positive Relationships*. Corio: Geelong Grammar School.

Norrish, J. M., Williams, P., O'Connor, M., & Robinson, J. (2013). An applied framework for positive education. *International Journal of wellbeing*. 3(2), 147-161. doi:10.5502/ijw.v3i2.2.

Ntoumanis, N. & Standage, M. (2009). Motivation in physical education classes: A self-determination theory perspective. http:// selfdeterminationtheory.org/SDT/documents/2009_ NtoumanisStandage_ TRE.pdf

O'Connell, B.H., O'Shea D. & Gallagher, S. (2017). Feeling Thanks and Saying Thanks: A Randomized Controlled Trial Examining If and How Socially Oriented Gratitude Journals Work. *Journal of Clinical Psychology.* 73(10):1280-1300. doi: 10.1002/jclp.22469.

Oettingen, G., Mayer, D., Sevincer, A., Stephens, E., Pak, H., & Hagenah, M. (2009). Mental contrasting and goal commitment: the mediating role of energization. *Personality and Psychology Bulletin.* 608-622.

Oxford Dictionary (2018). https://www.oxforddictionaries.com/

Park, N., & Peterson, C. (2006). Moral competence and character strengths among adolescents: The development and validation of the Values in Action Inventory of Strengths for Youth. *Journal of Adolescence.* 891-909.

Park, N., Peterson, C., & Seligman, M. (2004). Strengths of character and wellbeing. *Journal of Social and Clinical Psychology.* 603-619.

Pascual-Leone, A., Freitas, C., Oberman, L., Horvath, J.C., Halko, M., Eldaief, M., Bashir, S., Vernet, M., Shafi, M., Westover, B., Vahabzadeh-Hagh, A &, Rotenberg, A. (2011). Characterising brain cortical plasticity and network dynamics across the age-span in health and disease with TMS-EEG and TMS-fMRI. *Brain Topography.* 302-315.

Perestelo-Perez, L., Barraca, J., Peñate, W., Rivero-Santana, A. & Alvarez-Perez, Y. (2017). Mindfulness-based interventions for the treatment of depressive rumination: Systematic review and meta-analysis. *International Journal of Clinical and Health Psychology.* 17 (3): 282–95. doi:10.1016/j.ijchp.2017.07.004.

Peterson, C. & Park, N. (2003). Positive psychology as the evenhanded positive psychologist views it. *Psychological Inquiry.* 14, 141-146.

Peterson, C. & Park, N. (2009). Classifying and measuring strengths of character. In S. J. Lopez & C. R. Snyder (Eds.), *Oxford handbook of positive psychology*. (2nd ed.). (pp. 25–33). New York, NY: Oxford University Press.

Peterson, C., & Seligman, M. (2003). Character strengths before and after September 11. *Psychological Science.* 381-384.

Peterson, C., & Seligman, M. (2004). Character strengths and virtues: a handbook and classification. New York: Oxford University Press & Washington DC: *American Psychological Association.*

Pink, D. (2009.) *Drive. The Surprising Truth about what motivates us.* Riverhead Books, New York.

Plutchik, R. (1997). The circumplex as a general model of the structure of emotions and personality. *American Psychological Association.* pp. 17–45. doi:10.1037/10261-001. ISBN 1557983801.

Post, S.G. (2005) Altruism, happiness, and health: it's good to be good. *International Journal of Clinical and Health Psychology.* 12: 66. https://doi.org/10.1207/s15327558ijbm1202_4

Pressman S.D. & Cohen S. (2005). Does positive affect influence health? *Psychological Bulletin* 2005 Nov;131(6):925-971. doi: 10.1037/0033-2909.131.6.925.

PriceWaterhouseCoopers (2014): Creating a mentally healthy workplace Return on investment analysis (https://www.headsup.org.au/docs/default-source/resources/beyondblue_ workplaceroi_finalreport_may-2014.pdf)

Querstret, D. & Cropley, M. (2013). Assessing treatments used to reduce rumination and/or worry: A systematic review. *Clinical Psychology Review.* 33 (8): 996–1009.

Quora (2017) https://www.quora.com/Is-your-glass-half-empty-or-half-full

Radel, R., Sarrazin, P., Legrain, P., & Wild, T. C. (2010). Social contagion of motivation between teacher and student: Analyzing underlying processes. Journal of Educational Psychology, 102(3), 577-587.

Raj, P., Elizabeth, C.S. & Padmakumari, P. (2016). Mental health through forgiveness: Exploring the roots and benefits. *Cogent Psychology.* 3:1, DOI: 10.1080/23311908.2016.1153817.

Rath, T. (2007). *StrengthsFinder 2.0.* New York: Gallup Press.

Rath. T. (2013). *Eat Move Sleep: How Small Choices Lead to Big Changes.* New York, NY Missionday.

Rath, T. & Clifton, D. (2004). *How full is your bucket?* Gallup Press.

Rathunde, K. (2003). A comparison of Montessori and traditional middle schools: Motivation, quality of experience, and social context. *Namta Journal.* 28.3 (2003): 12-53.

ReachOut (2018). Wellbeing and Resilience https://au.reachout.com/articles/wellbeing – and-resilience

Redelmeier, D.A. & Tibshirani, R.J. (1999) Why cars in the next lane seem to go faster. *Nature* Vol 101 http://apps.usd.edu/coglab/schieber/psyc707/pdf/Redelmeier1999.pdf

Reivich, K. & Shatte, A. (2003). *The Resilience Factor.* R Wyler & Co.

Robertson, I.T., Cooper, C.L., Sarkar, M. & Curran, T. (2015). Resilience training in the workplace from 2003 to 2014: A systematic review. *Journal of Occupational and Organizational Psychology.* 88 (3): 533–562. doi:10.1111/joop.12120. ISSN 0963-1798.

Rogers, E. M. (2003). *Diffusion of Innovations* (5th ed.) New York, NY: Free Press.

Rohn, J. (2017): Wherever You Are, Be There. https://www.success.com/rohn-wherever-you -are-be-there/

Rosenthal, N. (2011). *Habit Formation*. Sussex Directories.

Rotter, J. (1966). Generalized expectancies for internal versus external control of reinforcements. Psychological Monographs: General and Applied, 80(1), 1-28.

Ryan, R.M. & Deci, E.L. (2000). Self-determination theory and the facilitation of intrinsic motivation, social development, and wellbeing. *American Psychologist.* 55 (1): 68–78. CiteSeerX 10.1.1.529.4370. doi:10.1037/0003-066X.55.1.68.

Ryan, R.M. & Deci, E.L. (2017). *Self-determination theory: Basic psychological needs in motivation, development, and wellness.* New York: Guilford Publishing.

Rye, M., Pargament, K.I., Ali, M., Beck, G., Dorff, E., Hallisey, C. & Williams, J.G. (2000). Religious perspectives on forgiveness. In M.E. McCullough, K.I. Pargament, and C.E.Thoresen (Eds.), *Forgiveness: Theory, research, and practice.* (pp. 17–40) New York, NY: Guilford.

Ryff, C. (1989) Happiness is everything, or is it? Explorations on the meaning of psychological wellbeing. *Journal of Personality and Social Psychology.* Vol 57(6), Dec 1989, 1069-1081 http://dx.doi.org/10.1037/0022-3514.57.6.1069

Salzberg, S. (1997) *Lovingkindness: The revolutionary art of happiness.* Boston: Shambhala.

Santos, M.E.C. (2018). The Japanese Secret to Finding One's Purpose is Forgetting Oneself. *The Ascent*. https://theascent.pub/the-japanese-secret-to-finding-ones-purpose-is-forgetting -oneself-6828edf58310.

Sapolsky, R. M. (2004). *Why Zebras Don't Get Ulcers*. 175 Fifth Ave, New York, N.Y.: St. Martins Press. pp. 37, 71, 92, 271.

Schuler, J. & Nakamura, J. (2013). Does flow experience lead to risk? How and for whom.

Applied Psychology, Health and Well Being. 2013 Nov;5(3):311-31. doi: 10.1111/aphw.12012.

Schunk, D.H., & Usher, E.L. (2012). Social cognitive theory and motivation. In R. M. Ryan (Ed.), *Oxford library of psychology. The Oxford handbook of human motivation*. (pp. 13-27). New York, NY, US: Oxford University Press.

Schwartz, B. (2004). *The Paradox of Choice: why more is less*. Harper Perennial.

Secker, J. (1998). Current conceptualizations of mental health and mental health promotion. (1). *Health Education Research*.13(1) p. 58.

Schwartz, B., & Ward, A. (2004). Doing Better but Feeling Worse: The Paradox of Choice. In P. A. Linley & S. Joseph (Eds.), *Positive psychology in practice*. (pp. 86-104). Hoboken, NJ, US: John Wiley & Sons Inc.

Segerstrom, S.C. (2014). Affect and self-rated health: A dynamic approach with older adults. *Health Psychology*. 33, 720–728.

Seligman, M. (2002). *Authentic Happiness*. New York: Free Press.

Seligman, M. (2011). *Flourish: a visionary new understanding of happiness and wellbeing*. New York: Simon & Schuster.

Seligman, M. & Csikszentmihalyi, M. (2000) Positive Psychology: An introduction. *American Psychologist.* 55, 5-14.

Seligman, M., & Csikszentmihalyi, M. (2014). *Positive psychology: An introduction.* (pp. 279-298). Springer Netherlands.

Seligman, M., Steen, T., & Peterson, C. (2005). Positive Psychology Progress: Empirical Validation of Interventions. *American psychologist.* 2005 – doi.apa.org

Semple, J., Lee, R. & Miller, F.l. (2006). Mindfulness-based cognitive therapy for children. In *Mindfulness-based treatment approaches: Clinician's guide to evidence base and applications.* Elsevier, Editor: Ruth A. Baer, pp.143-166.

Sheldon, K.M., Abad, N., Ferguson, Y., Gunz, A., Houser-Marko, L., Nichols, C.P. & Lyubomirsky, S. (2010). Persistent pursuit of need-satisfying goals leads to increased happiness: A 6-month experimental longitudinal study. *Motivation and Emotion.* 34(1), 39-48.

Siefert, C., & Patalano, A. (2001). Opportunism in memory: preparing for chance encounters. *Current Directions in Psychological Science.* 198-201.

Sin, N.L. & Lyubomirsky, S. (2009). Enhancing Well-Being and Alleviating Depressive Symptoms with Positive Psychology Interventions: A Practice-Friendly Meta-Analysis. *Journal of Clinical Psychology.* 65 (5):467–487. doi:10.1002/jclp.

Sinek, Simon (2011) *Start with Why.* Penguin Books Ltd.

Slade, T., Johnston, A., Teesson, M., Whiteford, H., Burgess, P. & Pirkis, J. (2009). *The Mental Health of Australians 2: Report on the 2007 National Survey of Mental Health and wellbeing.* Canberra: Department of Health and Ageing.

Smiling Mind (n.d.) https://www.youtube.com/channel/UCSP__8_QEFYdi0gY2F3CXfA

Smith, C., & Davidson, H. (2014). *The Paradox of Generosity: Giving We Receive, Grasping We Lose*. New York: Oxford University Press.

Smith, E, E. (2017). *The Power of Meaning: Crafting a Life That Matters*. Random House, UK.

Snel, E. (2013). *Sitting Still Like a Frog, Mindfulness Exercises for Kids (and their Parents)*. Shambhala, Boston & London.

Srinivasan, T. S. (2015). *The 5 Founding Fathers and A History of Positive Psychology*. https://positivepsychologyprogram.com/founding-fathers/

Stajkovic, A.D., Locke, E.A. & Blair, E.S. (2006). A first examination of the relationships between primed subconscious goals, assigned conscious goals, and task performance. *Journal of Applied Psychology*. 91 (5): 1172–1180. doi:10.1037/0021-9010.91.5.1172. PMID 16953778.

Staw, B., Sutton, R., & Pelled, L. (1994). Employee positive emotions and favourable outcomes at the workplace. *Organisational Science*. 51-71.

Steger, M. F., & Frazier, P. (2005). Meaning in life: One link in the chain from religion to wellbeing. Journal of Counseling Psychology. 52, 574–582.

Steger, M.F., Kashdan, T.B., & Oishi, S. (2008). Being good by doing good: Daily eudaimonic activity and wellbeing. *Journal of Research in Personality*. 42, 22–42.

Sternberg, R. (1998). *In Search of the Human Mind* 2nd Ed. Harcourt, Brace p 542.

Stewart, D., Sun, J., Patterson, C., Lemerle, K. & Hardie, M. (2004). *Promoting and Building Resilience in Primary School Communities: Evidence from a Comprehensive 'Health Promoting School' Approach.* Centre for Health Research, School of Public Health, Queensland University of Technology. https://eprints.qut.edu.au/1281/1/IJMHP.pdf

Street, H., O'Connor, M & Robinson, H. (2007). Depression in older adults: Exploring the relationship between goal setting and physical health. *International Journal of Geriatric Psychiatry.* 22: 1115-1119.

Suldo, S., Thalji, A., & Ferron, J. (2011). Longitudinal academic outcomes predicted by early adolescents' subjective wellbeing, psychopathology and mental health status yielded from a dual factor model. *Journal of Positive Psychology.* 17-30.

Sullivan, M.D. (2003). Hope and hopelessness at the end of life. *American Journal of Geriatric Psychiatry.* 11(4):393-405.)

Syme, S.L. (1998). Mastering the control factor. *The Health Report, ABC Radio.* Health Report transcript 9.11.1998. www.abc.net.au/rn

Syme, S.L. & Balfour, J.L. (1997). Explaining inequalities in coronary heart disease. *Lancet.* 350(9073):231-2.

Tan, Chade-Meng (2012). *Search Inside Yourself, Increase productivity, creativity and happiness.* HarperCollins, London.

Tanasescu, M., Leitzmann, M.F., Rimm, E.B., Willett, W.C., Stampfer, J.J. & Hu, F.B. (2002). Exercise type and intensity in relation to coronary heart disease in men. *Journal of the American Medical Association.* 288:1994-2000.

Tang, Y., Leve, L.D. (2015). A translational neuroscience perspective on mindfulness meditation as a prevention strategy. *Translational Behavioral*

Medicine. 6 (1): 63–72. doi:10.1007/s13142-015-0360-x. PMC 4807201. PMID 27012254.

Tangney, J., Fee, R., Reinsmith, C., Boone, A. L. & Lee, N. (1999). Assessing individual differences in the propensity to forgive. Paper presented at the annual meeting of the American Psychological Association, Boston, MA.

Tedeshi, R.G., & Calhoun, L.G. (2004). Posttraumatic Growth: Conceptual Foundation and Empirical Evidence. Philadelphia, PA: Lawrence Erlbaum Associates.

Thune, I. & Lund, E. (1997). The influence of physical activity on lung cancer risk. *International Journal of Cancer.* 70: 57-62.

Timpano, K.R.; Schmidt, N.B. (2013). The relationship between self control deficits and hoarding: A multimethod investigation across three samples. *The Journal of Abnormal Psychology.* 122 (1): 13–25. doi:10.1037/a0029760.

Toffler, A. (1970) *Future Shock.* Random House.

Tomlinson E.R., Yousaf, O., Vitterso, A.D. & Jones, L. (2018). Dispositional mindfulness and psychological health: a systematic review. *Mindfulness.* 9 (1): 23–43. doi:10.1007/s12671-017-0762-6. PMC 5770488. PMID 29387263.

Tov, W. & Diener, E.F. (2013., Subjective Well-Being. *Research Collection School of Social Sciences.* Paper 1395. http://ink.library.sju.edu.sg/soss_research/1395

Townsend, M., Kladder, V., Ayele H., & Mulligan, T. (2002). Systematic review of clinical trials examining the effects of religion on health. *Southern Medical Journal.* 95(12):1429-34.

Truempy, K. (2014) *The Positive Psychology Podcast.* https://www.stitcher.com/podcast /kristen-truempy/ the-positive – psychology-podcast.

Trustees of the University of Pennsylvania, The. (2018). *Authentic Happiness* https://www.authentichappiness.sas.upenn.edu/user/login?destination=node/463

Tsvetkova, M., & Macy, M. (2014). *The Social Contagion of Generosity.* PLoS ONE.

Van Ryzin, M.J., Gravely, A.A. & Roseth, C.J. (2009). Autonomy, belongingness, and engagement in school as contributors to adolescent psychological wellbeing. *Journal of Youth and Adolescence.* 38(1):1-12. doi: 10.1007/s10964-007-9257-4.

Vasalampi, K., Salmela-Aro, J. & Nurmi, J.E. (2009). Adolescents' Self-Concordance, School Engagement, and Burnout Predict Their Educational Trajectories. *European Psychologist.* 14(4).

VIA Institute on Character (2019) http://www.viacharacter.org/www/#

Warneken, F., Chen, F. & Tomasello, M. (2006). Cooperative activities in young children and chimpanzees. *Child development.* 77(3), pp.640-663.

Watkins, E. (2015). Psychological treatment of depressive rumination. *Current Opinion in Psychology.* 4: 32–36. http://www.academia.edu/34020644/Psychological_Treatment_of_ Depressive_Rumination

Wentzell, K.R. & Caldwell, K. (1997). Friendships, Peer Acceptance, and Group Membership: Relations to Academic Achievement in Middle School. *Child Development.* Vol. 68, No. 6. 1198-1209.

WHO (2004). Promoting mental health: Concepts, emerging evidence, practice (summary report). Geneva: World Health Organization.

WHO (2011). Health promoting schools. http://www.who.int/school_youth_health/gshi/ hps/en/index.html

WHO (2018a). Constitution of WHO https://www.who.int/about/mission/en/

WHO (2018b.) Adolescent Mental Health http://www.who.int/news-room/fact-sheets/detail/adolescent -mental-health

Wigfield, A., Guthrie, J.T., Tonks, S. & Perencevich, K.C. (2004). Children's motivation for reading: Domain specificity and instructional influences. *Journal of Educational Research.* 97 (6): 299–309. doi:10.3200/joer.97.6.299-310.

Wolin, S.J. & Wolin, S. (2010). *The Resilient Self: How Survivors of Troubled Families Rise Above Adversity.* Random House Publishing Group. ISBN 978-0-307-75687-9.

Wood, A.M., Froh, J.J., & Geraghty, A.W. (2010). Gratitude and wellbeing: A review and theoretical integration. *Clinical Psychology Review* https://greatergood.berkeley.edu/pdfs/GratitudePDFs/2Wood-GratitudeWell-BeingReview.pdf

Wood, W., Quinn, J., & Kashy, D. (2002). Habits in Everyday Life: The Thought and Feel of Action. *Journal of Personality and Social Psychology.* 1281–1297.

Yates, T.M., Egeland, B., & Sroufe, L.A. (2003). Rethinking resilience: A developmental process perspective. pp. 234–256 in S. S. Luthar (Ed.), *Resilience and vulnerability: Adaptation in the context of childhood adversities.* New York: Cambridge University Press, ISBN 0521001617.

Zhang, J.W., Piff, P.K. & Iyer, R. An occasion for unselfing: Beautiful nature leads to prosociality. *Journal of Environmental Psychology.* 2014;37:61-72. doi: 10.1016/j.jenvp.2013.11.008.

Praise For Unleashing Personal Potential

At Unleashing Personal Potential (UPP), we work with schools who are serious about making a positive change and helping their students to learn, live and lead better. It is our honour to call them our partners.

Testimonials from some of our school partners are included below. For more testimonials from our school partners, please refer to http://www. unleashingpersonalpotential.com.au/

If you're serious about helping students learn, live and lead better, contact admin@unleashingpersonalpotential.com.au and we can discuss the best approach for UPP to work with your school.

PRIMARY SCHOOLS

"Amazing day and really engaging. Students and teachers really enjoyed it." Teacher- Coomera Rivers State School.

"The best leadership program I have seen." Religious Education Leader, Our Lady of the Rosary, Kyneton, Melbourne.

"Yesterday was fantastic and Hogan was extraordinary. The students were very engaged and enthusiastic about what they learnt. I thought the structure of the day was very good. I'm glad I took the risk in trying something new. It paid off!" Teacher- Ashburton Primary School.

WOW! What a brilliant day! Pete had the kids attention and they were motivated and fully engaged all day. Thanks for such a great service. Principal- St Mary MacKillop Primary School, Keilor Downs.

"Excellent day! Students engaged 100% of the time." Teacher- Musgrave Hill State School.

"Fun, professional, very pertinent, accessible." Teacher- Mooloolaba State School.

"We were very impressed with the day. The timing was perfect and the topics were very appropriate. The children enjoyed the day and related well to the presenters. We look forward to enjoying the experience at the same time next year" Teacher- MacKillop Catholic Primary, Birkdale.

SECONDARY SCHOOLS

"Dynamic, powerful, engaging, relevant." Middle School Coordinator- Brigidine College, Indooroopilly.

"Engaging, interesting and expertly managed session." Teacher- Mt Maria College.

"UPP are highly professional in their approach, facilitating a leadership day with our College that uses theory and practical activities to engage and inspire our students to make an impact as College leaders in their senior year." Head of Students- Marist College, Ashgrove.

"Fantastic. Excellent to see all students actively participating. Students were highly engaged and had a lot to take away." Teacher- Toogoolawah State High School.

"This presentation was excellent and very engaging. Had the right amount of humour. The stories from our presenters had a massive impact." House Dean- St Patrick's College, Shorncliffe.

"We were extremely impressed with the presentation. The students were highly engaged and I felt that the session was a valuable one with a message that the students needed to hear. I don't think it would hurt for the whole school to hear a similar message delivered that well every term. A great presentation. I was in agreement with all points. It was one of the most significant moments of the year. Empathy, consideration, social skills, emotional intelligence. I loved it! He was a character I could relate to." Teacher- Lowood State High School.

"Immediately took all of our students out of their comfort zone, challenging them physically, emotionally and intellectually. Presenters very quickly established great rapport and respect. Awesome." Year Coordinator- Yeppoon State High School.

"An outstanding experience of leadership, through connection, activity, conversation, engagement and influence." Assistant Principal (Students)- Lourdes Hill College.

"This is the best program I have seen in many years in this job. Well presented, energetic, meaningful with clear messages. Appropriate activities that allowed leadership and teamwork to be shown. Excellent." Head of House- Marist College, Ashgrove.

"Fantastic day with a great message. All students should experience this." Teacher- Elanora State High School.

THRIVE ONLINE LESSON MODULES

"The UPP online modules and lesson plans have made the teachers jobs easier, with resources and introductory activities that are not only engaging, but extremely relevant." Year Coordinator- Macgregor State High School.

"The THRIVE resources are a wonderful introduction to vital concepts such as growth mindset, grit and wellbeing. The resources are easy to access and the teachers find them very dynamic and easy to interact with. The feedback from our students has also been extremely positive." Positive Education & Wellbeing Coordinator- Varsity College.

TEACHER PROFESSIONAL DEVELOPMENT

"Best PD I've ever attended in 7 years of teaching. The entire day was useful. A fantastic presentation!" Teacher- St Clare's Primary School, Townsville.

"It was fantastic. Great ideas, practical, engaging. Great presenter." Head of Clan- The Springfield Anglican College.

"A fantastic presentation that provides teachers with the tools to help students be the best they can be." Deputy Principal- Murrumba State Secondary College.

"Thoroughly engaging and enlightening. Great presentation." Deputy Principal- Shailer Park State High School.

"A clear, steamlined presentation with key topics that are very relevant to how we might start an action plan and change school culture." Deputy Principal- Burpengary State School.

"Engaging presentation, all very relevant. Great use of analogies and examples for clarity. Activities were well placed throughout." Teacher-Brigidine College.

"One of the best PD sessions that our whole staff have ever experienced."

Principal, St Andrews Catholic School, Ferny Grove.

"Well presented, informative, engaging sessions, which gave tangible actions to help deliver the content." Teacher- Coolum State High School.